Motor
Neuron
Disease

Project Development Manager: Louise Cook
Project Manager: Scott Millar
Design: Andy Chapman
Illustrations Manager: Mick Ruddy

Motor Neuron Disease

Edited by

Ralph W Kuncl MD, PhD

Professor of Neurology
Vice Provost, Johns Hopkins University
Baltimore, USA

W.B. SAUNDERS

London • Edinburgh • New York • Philadelphia • St Louis • Sydney • Toronto 2002

WB SAUNDERS
An imprint of Elsevier Science Limited

© 2002, Elsevier Science Limited. All rights reserved

 is a registered trademark of
Elsevier Science Limited

First published 2002

ISBN 0–7020–2528–3

British Library Cataloguing in Publication Data
A catalogue record for this book is available from the British Library

Library of Congress Cataloging in Publication Data
A catalog record for this book is available from the Library of Congress

Note
Medical knowledge is constantly changing. As new information becomes
available, changes in treatment, procedures, equipment and the use of
drugs become necessary. The authors and the publishers have taken care to
ensure that the information given in this text is accurate and up to date.
However, readers are strongly advised to confirm that the information,
especially with regard to drug usage, complies with the latest legislation
and standards of practice.

Existing UK nomenclature is changing to the system of Recommended
International Nonproprietary Names (rINNs). Until the UK names are no
longer in use, these more familiar names are used in this book in preference
to rINNs, details of which may be obtained from the British National
Formulary.

The
publisher's
policy is to use
paper manufactured
from sustainable forests

Printed by RDC Group in China

Contents

Contributors

Frank Baldino
Chairman and Chief Executive Officer
Cephalon, Inc.
West Chester, PA
USA

Patricia Casey
Occupational Therapist
Neurological Disorders Program
North Western University Medical
  School
Chicago, IL
USA

Thomas Crawford
Associate Professor of Neurology
  and Pediatrics
Johns Hopkins Hospital
Department of Neurology
Baltimore, Maryland
USA

Joy Desai
The Royal London Hospital
Department of Neurology
London
United Kingdom

Andrew Eisen
Vancouver General Hospital
Vancouver, British Columbia
Canada

John Farah
Vice President, Worldwide Business
  Development
Cephalon, Inc.
West Chester, PA
USA

Jaques Hugon
Professor of Cell Biology, Histology
  and Neurology
Faculty of Medicine

Department of Anatomy
Hong Kong

Ralph Kuncl
Provost and Professor of Biology
Bryn Mawr College
Bryn Mawr, PA
USA

Formerly Vice Provost and Professor
  of Neurology, Johns Hopkins
  University

Albert Ludolph
Professor and Chair of Neurology
University of Ulm
Department of Neurology
Ulm, Germany

Judith Richman
Neuromuscular Nurse Clinician
Rush-Presbyterian – St Luke's
  Medical Center
Chicago, IL
USA

Wim Robberecht
Professor of Neurology
University Hospital Gastnuisberg
Department of Neurology
Belgium

Pamela Shaw
Wellcome Senior Fellow in Clinical
  Science
Royal Victoria Infirmary
Newcastle Upon Tyne
United Kingdom

Michael Swash
Professor of Neurology
Barts and the London School of
  Medicine
Department of Neurology
London
United Kingdom

Preface

One may well ask why we need 'yet another book on motor neuron disease' now, and why we need a book of this scope. Volumes on motor neuron disorders are appearing at the rate of several per year, rather than the one-every-seven-years typical of the 1960s through 1980s. Motor neuron diseases are a frontier in neurology and neuroscience. Knowledge is changing at a much faster rate than in any previous decade. The SOD-1 mutation in familial ALS was reported in 1993, the SMN mutation of spinal muscular atrophy in 1995, and a host of other important pathophysiological mechanisms have been investigated in depth. One need only compare the increasing number of journal articles on motor neuron diseases in three leading international neurology journals (*Annals of Neurology, Journal of Neurology, Neurosurgery and Psychiatry,* and *Neurology*) in 1978, 1988, and 1998 to see the explosion in knowledge and interest. In that era, the number of entries increased eight fold from 9 to 41 to 73 per year. The diseases even spawned a new journal in 1999, *Amyotrophic Lateral Sclerosis and Other Motor Neuron Disorders*, as the official publication of the World Federation of Neurology Group on Motor Neuron Diseases. That the *pubmed* database now includes 14,000 Journal articles related to motor neuron diseases further indicates the information boom.

Therapy has also changed dramatically. No approved, disease-modifying therapy existed before 1995, when riluzole was marketed. The approval of insulin-like growth factor I for ALS continues to be uncertain in the USA, despite one positive placebo-controlled multicenter trial and a second trial showing a trend in the same direction but which missed statistical significance (IGF-I is available only in Japan for treatment of dwarfism). A host of other neurotrophic factors and anti-glutamatergic drugs are under active study. Gabapentin, at first seemingly promising, failed in a larger multicenter trial. Stem cell approaches and gene-based therapies are the near future. More than a dozen clinical trials for ALS are under way at any one time, whereas before 1980 published trials were rare. This is amazing, as a single clinical trial may cost between $1 million and $100 million. ALS has become a 'model' neurodegenerative disease for the pharmaceutical industry because of its predictability, the quasi-linearity of the decline in strength, and the directness of possible outcome measures, with the hope that successful treatments may find applicability generally in other neurodegenerations or traumatic disorders of the CNS. A nonscientific approach to ALS therapy persists, and it is interesting that the weakly anti-oxidant vitamin E is now taken ubiquitously for sporadic ALS despite a quite limited rationale 60 years after it was Lou Gehrig's sole 'anti-aging' therapy for ALS.

Therefore, because of the explosion of knowledge and the therapeutic possibilities, this book is aimed at the neurological clinician in all settings, both academic and practice. A book of this scope is designed for the clinician who wants to be at the cutting edge of the scientific understanding of motor neuron disease and up to date on the clinical art. It attempts to answer the following questions for clinicians of all types (broadly defined to include physicians, nurses, physician's assistants, nurse practitioners, and therapists) who see patients with motor neuron disorders:

- What are the current accepted diagnostic criteria for ALS? What essential tests must I perform when I see a patient suspected of having ALS? What can mistaken diagnoses teach me about differential diagnosis and my own diagnostic approach?
- There are many theories of pathogenesis, but which have the most support and how can I synthesize them all? Is ALS likely to have multiple causes?
- When should I test for SOD-1 mutations in affected patients and their relatives, and what do I do with the information? Are there any new gene defects linked with ALS? How do I make sense of the complicated genetics of SMN mutations in SMA? Has modern genetics changed the diagnostic criteria for SMA?
- Is SMA still hopeless or are there new treatments on the horizon?
- Since the advent of the Internet, my patients seem to know more than I do about new therapies. What are the real scientific bases for what's being offered now and what's about to come out in the next year or two?
- What do I do when there's 'nothing to do', in order to support my patient and manage the symptomatic care?
- Clinical trials seem to abound in ALS. Why are they all designed differently? In the riluzole era, what are the issues of trial size, best outcome measures, need for placebo controls? Tell me what I need to know to advise my patients about participation and advocate for them. What are the pharmaceutical industry's perspectives on the difficulty in bringing promising drugs to market quickly for a terrible fatal, but 'orphan', disease?
- Look into the crystal ball; what is down the line for ALS and SMA?

What a book of this scope cannot do is explore encyclopedically the many interesting details of all the ongoing cellular and molecular aspects of each pathophysiological hypothesis about motor neuron diseases, except where they impact current and immediate future therapy. That is left to other books and other times. It also cannot deal in detail with *every* motor neuron disease, but emphasizes the three most common ones – sporadic ALS, familial ALS, and childhood SMA – to the near exclusion of polio, post-polio amyotrophy, Kennedy's spinobulbar muscular atrophy, juvenile familial ALS, distal spinal muscular atrophy, and many other rare forms.

Knowledge continues to change rapidly, so a book is merely a slice in time. The reader is encouraged to consider the many ways of keeping up in the Internet era by consulting the following websites and related resources:

- The World Federation of Neurology's Research Group on Motor Neuron Diseases maintains a cooperative, international website. It contains the El Escorial/Arlie House Criteria, 1998 (a consensus document detailing up-to-date diagnostic criteria). *www.wfnals.org*
- The World Alliance of Neuromuscular Disorder Associations (WANDA) site contains a comprehensive listing of how to contact most of the world's agencies devoted to muscular dystrophies and motor neuron diseases. *www.w-a-n-d-a.org*

- Muscular Dystrophy Associations exist in many countries. Besides those listed in WANDA (above), the largest that also focus on amyotrophic lateral sclerosis or spinal muscular atrophy are:

  United Kingdom (Muscular Dystrophy Campaign) – *www.muscular-dystrophy.org*

  United States (Muscular Dystrophy Association) – *www.mdausa.org* (which publishes an ALS Newsletter at *www.mdausa.org/publications/als/index.html*)

- Associations focused on amyotrophic lateral sclerosis, motor neuron disease, or spinal muscular atrophy also have worldwide scope:

  United Kingdom (Amyotrophic Lateral Sclerosis/Motor Neuron Disease Alliance) – *www.alsmndalliance.org*

  United States (Amyotrophic Lateral Sclerosis Association) – *www.alsa.org* (Families of Spinal Muscular Atrophy) – *www.fsma.org*

Innumerable other sites devoted to motor neuron diseases offer information not vetted by any authority, which 'information' the Internet user should both enjoy and beware!

RWK

Acknowledgements

The author wishes to acknowledge the contributions of the following groups for their generous support of research on ALS over the years: The Dino and Wendy Fabbri Fund for Neuromuscular Research, the Sue Mullen Fund, the Gail Rupertus Fund, the Jay Slotkin Fund, the Mid-Atlantic Classic Fund, the Cal Ripken Jr./Lou Gehrig Fund for Neuromuscular Disease, the Muscular Dystrophy Association (USA), and the National Institute of Neurological Disorders and Stroke.

To
Parker and Margaux

CHAPTER 1

Essentials of diagnosis

Joy Desai and Michael Swash

Introduction

The nomenclature of the adult-onset disorders of the motor system can be confusing (Table 1.1). This confusion reflects ignorance of the underlying causes of these syndromes. Current terminology is based on clinical or pathological descriptions of the syndromes themselves rather than basic mechanisms. This confusion in terminology can be resolved by appreciation of the historical development of the concept of anterior horn cell disease as a cause of muscle wasting.

Progressive muscular wasting was a clinical syndrome well known to physicians in the early nineteenth century. The term *progressive muscular atrophy* was used by Aran (1850), who believed this syndrome was a muscular

Table 1.1 Nomenclature of disorders of the motor system

Idiopathic motor neuron diseases
- Amyotrophic lateral sclerosis (ALS)
- Progressive bulbar palsy (PBP)
- Progressive muscular atrophy (PMA)
- Primary lateral sclerosis (PLS)
- Familial amyotrophic lateral sclerosis (FALS)
- Juvenile amyotrophic lateral sclerosis (JALS)
- Madras motor neuron disease
- Monomelic motor neuron disease (amyotrophy)

Toxin-related motor neuron diseases
- Lathyrism
- Konzo
- Guamanian ALS

Motor disorders resembling motor neuron disease
- Adult-onset proximal spinal muscular atrophy
- X-linked bulbospinal neuronopathy
- Radiation myelopathy
- Paraneoplastic motor neuron disease
- Motor disorders associated with thyroid and parathyroid disease
- Hexosaminidase deficiency
- Electric shock and lightning injuries
- Postpolio syndrome (amyotrophy)
- Paraproteinemia
- Heavy metal intoxication: lead, mercury
- Multifocal motor neuropathy

disorder. Duchenne (1849) also gave a description of this disorder. Bell, supported by Cruveilhier (1853), who noted the thinness of the anterior spinal roots, regarded progressive muscular atrophy as a myelopathic disorder, whereas Aran and Duchenne favored a muscular cause. Degeneration of the anterior cells in the grey matter of the spinal cord was recognized independently by Luys (1860) in Paris, and by Lockhart Clarke in London. Charcot (1869) brought together these observations by studying the clinical and pathological features of the disease and described the involvement of the corticospinal tract. Charcot proposed the term *amyotrophic lateral sclerosis. Progressive bulbar palsy* was described by Duchenne (1860). Charcot and Joffroy (1869) recognized its relationship to amyotrophic lateral sclerosis when loss of motor neurons was noted in the bulbar motor nuclei in pathological studies at the Hôpital Salpêtrière. Pure syndromes of myelopathic weakness without muscular atrophy, e.g. *primary lateral sclerosis* as described by Spiller (1904), are rare and until recently have always been regarded as related to the core syndrome of *amyotrophic lateral sclerosis*.

The term *motor neuron disease* was introduced by Brain (1962) in recognition of the relation between the syndromes of progressive muscular atrophy, amyotrophic lateral sclerosis and progressive bulbar palsy, as shown by the clinical variation of involvement of upper and lower motor neurons and by the topography of the muscular wasting. This term has become commonly used in the UK, although Charcot's designation *amyotrophic lateral sclerosis* is preferred in French-speaking countries and the United States, where it has come to specify the combination of lower and upper motor neuron disease.

Rowland (1982) recognised the utility of the term motor neuron disease (MND) in describing the whole clinical syndrome but stressed the importance of retaining the general usage of the term *motor neuron diseases* (plural) to describe all the diseases of the anterior horn cells and motor system, including the inherited spinal muscular atrophies that are clinically and pathologically distinct from MND itself.

In this chapter the term *motor neuron disease* (MND, used in the singular form) will be synonymous with the term *amyotrophic lateral sclerosis* (ALS). The term *motor neuron diseases* (plural) will apply to the broad category of disorders of the anterior horn cell, cortical Betz cells, and the corticospinal tracts.

Characteristic clinical features of motor neuron diseases

Amyotrophic lateral sclerosis

Amyotrophic lateral sclerosis (ALS) is a relentlessly progressive, fatal disorder of the nervous system that results from the degeneration of upper and lower motor neurons. The pathophysiological process is typically restricted to the cortical Betz cells, the corticospinal tracts, certain cranial motor neurons in the brainstem and the neurons in the ventral horn of the spinal cord. These different parts of the neuraxis are involved simultaneously in varying severity and combination. This results in a characteristic clinical profile of symptoms and signs. Rarely, and late in the course of the disease process, extrapyramidal and even spinocerebellar pathways may be involved (Swash et al., 1988). A frontal type of dementia may also develop in rare cases (Neary et al., 1990).

The clinical features of ALS depend on its severity and variable permutations of combined upper and lower motor neuron dysfunction affecting the susceptible parts of the neuraxis.

- The symptoms of lower motor neuron dysfunction are weakness, cramps, incoordination and fatigue, while its physical signs are the presence of weakness, atrophy, fasciculations, hypotonia and suppression of deep tendon reflexes (Table 1.2).
- The symptoms of upper motor neuron dysfunction are stiffness and slowing, incoordination, and weakness, while the corresponding physical signs are the presence of spasticity, brisk deep tendon reflexes and abnormal reflexes, especially the Babinski and Hoffman signs (Table 1.3).

Depending on the site of onset, the extent of involvement of the neuraxis in the disease process, and the stage of the disease, these symptoms and signs are present in varying combinations.

An asymmetric, distal onset is the most common mode of presentation of ALS. The patient typically complains of tripping, difficulty negotiating curbs, dragging of a foot, and ultimately more diffuse weakness of the leg. Difficulty with buttoning clothes, turning keys in doors, picking up objects, twisting off jar caps or simply poor coordination while performing fine movements are the symptoms of involvement of the upper limbs. Occasionally, proximal arm muscles may be involved early in the illness. Weakness may not be detected by

Table 1.2 Clinical features of lower motor neuron dysfunction

Symptoms
- Weakness
- Cramps
- Twitching of muscles
- Incoordination
- Fatigue

Signs
- Weakness
- Atrophy
- Fasciculations
- Suppression of reflexes
- Hypotonia

Table 1.3 Clinical features of upper motor neuron dysfunction

Symptoms
- Stiffness
- Slowing
- Incoordination
- Weakness

Signs
- Spasticity
- Brisk reflexes
- Babinski and Hoffman signs
- Weakness

manual muscle testing until 50% of motor neurons have died (Beasley, 1961). Several additional variables such as mood, affect, patient motivation, and general level of fatigue may affect measurement of strength. In spite of the loss of lower motor neuron function, unless muscles are grossly weak, the performance of repetitive movements like cycling or rhythmic tapping is normal since motor control and sensory input from superficial and deep sensation are preserved. Some patients note otherwise asymptomatic wasting of the muscles of the dorsum of the hand. Many patients complain of 'twitching of muscles' or 'muscle shaking' (especially on direct questioning). These symptoms reflect the presence of fasciculations, a sign almost universally noted in ALS though not at all specific to the disorder. Although 'cramps' or 'spasms' are frequent, as in other denervating diseases, the absence of overt sensory dysfunction, sphincter dysfunction, and oculomotor dysfunction serves to distinguish ALS from other disorders of the lower motor neuron.

Bulbar involvement in ALS often presents with subtle changes in speech and occasional difficulty in swallowing fluids progressing to overt dysarthria, hypophonia, dysphagia, drooling of saliva and rarely even nasal regurgitation. Patients present with a pseudobulbar palsy characterized by spastic dysarthria, dysphagia and spontaneous outbursts of laughter and crying known as 'pseudobulbar affect'. Neurological evaluation reveals a brisk jaw jerk, slow, spastic tongue movements, and an exaggerated gag reflex. Bulbar dysfunction is less often predominantly lower motor neuron in origin. A wasted, fasciculating tongue, and diminished palatal movements accompany limb weakness in these patients, a feature particularly important in the diagnosis of ALS.

Patients with predominant upper limb or bulbar involvement often have weak respiratory muscles. This results in breathlessness on minimal exertion and, especially when there is diaphragmatic weakness, on lying supine. Poor nocturnal sleep, excessive daytime sleepiness, headaches on awakening, and excessive nocturnal sweating are features of early respiratory failure. Involvement of the respiratory musculature is often accompanied by activation of the accessory muscles of respiration during normal breathing, poor cough, and an abnormal 'sniff test' on neurological assessment. This may progress to frank respiratory failure requiring ventilatory assistance.

ALS begins with limb involvement in 65–80% of patients, while bulbar onset is noted in 20–25% (Lawyer and Netsky, 1953; Vejjajiva et al., 1967; Jablecki et al., 1989). The disease invariably progresses with time, and symptoms and signs spread to involve contiguous body parts (Tan et al., 1988). EMG changes may antedate clinical weakness and atrophy, suggesting that symptom accrual is a function of the balance between denervation and reinnervation in a region after initiation of the disease process (Swash and Ingram, 1988). The spread of the disease process to contiguous spinal segments within the corresponding spinal cord results in clinical and electrophysiological evidence of involvement of muscles within the corresponding spinal regions. This may sometimes cause diagnostic confusion with other diseases, particularly when root involvement is suspected (see Chapter 2) and must surely bear on pathophysiological mechanisms (Chapter 3). Within individual spinal segments, anterior horn cell loss is random (Swash et al., 1986). Progressive anterior horn cell loss results in increasing disability ultimately leading to a bedbound state. In contrast to other paralyzing neurological conditions, bedsores are rare in ALS, in spite of the patient being bedbound. Perhaps this is because sensation is spared in ALS. The usual course of ALS is relentlessly progressive, with death by three years in about half of patients (Mulder and Howard, 1976).

A small proportion of patients with ALS may develop personality and behavioral change. Cognitive assessment reveals impairment in planning ability, execution of strategies and ability to perform complex sequential tasks occasionally associated with frontal lobe release signs (Neary et al., 1990). Although dementia is not a characteristic feature of ALS, these features reflect the involvement of the frontal lobes in the disease process (Abrahams et al., 1996; Jackson et al., 1996). These features are more common in patients with bulbar involvement (Abrahams et al., 1997).

Rarely, some patients exhibit parkinsonian features in addition to the characteristic motor signs of ALS (Qureshi et al., 1996).

Progressive bulbar palsy

Progressive bulbar palsy (PBP) denotes a progressive disease presenting with bulbar dysfunction due to destruction of motor neurons in the brainstem. Sometimes this syndrome includes evidence of upper motor neuron dysfunction. Historically, it has been considered a 'bulbar' form of ALS/MND. Clinically the disorder has to be differentiated from conditions with a similar initial presentation, e.g. subcortical arteriosclerotic leukoencephalopathy or Binswanger's disease, Steele–Richardson–Olszewski syndrome, foramen magnum tumors, clivus chordomas, and polyneuritis cranialis.

Progressive muscular atrophy

Progressive muscular atrophy (PMA) refers to motor neuron disease presenting with weakness and wasting of muscles of the limb and trunk muscles without evidence of upper motor neuron dysfunction. This condition may mimic adult onset proximal spinal muscular atrophy (SMA). The more rapid progression, and the later development of brisk reflexes, may assist in differentiating PMA from SMA, since in SMA the tendon reflexes are usually reduced, and the plantar responses are always flexor.

Primary lateral sclerosis

Primary lateral sclerosis (PLS) typically presents with a slowly progressive spastic gait disorder. Over months or years, the upper limbs are involved and in most patients a pseudobulbar syndrome develops. Hyperreflexia, and Babinski and Hoffman signs are characteristic features, whereas lower motor neuron dysfunction and sphincter dysfunction are absent. The clinical course and survival are much longer than ALS of Charcot type. Based on clinical, radiological and pathological studies (Younger et al., 1988; Pringle et al., 1992) diagnostic criteria have been laid down (Table 1.4). PLS may be a paraneoplastic manifestation of breast carcinoma (Forsyth et al., 1997). PLS is a very rare disorder; Pringle et al., were able to review only 23 published cases in 1992. Part of the nosological problem with PLS as a diagnosis is that if lower

Table 1.4 Proposed diagnostic criteria for PLS (Pringle et al. 1992)

Clinical
1. Insidious onset of spastic paraparesis, usually beginning in lower extremities but occasionally bulbar or upper extremities
2. Adult onset, usually fifth decade or later
3. Absence of family history
4. Gradually progressive course (i.e. not step-like)
5. Duration > 3 years
6. Clinical findings limited to those associated with corticospinal dysfunction
7. Symmetrical distribution, ultimately developing severe spastic spinobulbar paresis

Laboratory
1. Normal serum chemistry including normal vitamin B_{12} levels
2. Negative serologic tests for syphilis (in endemic areas negative Lyme and HTLV-1 serology)
3. Normal CSF parameters, including absence of oligoclonal bands
4. Absent denervation potentials on EMG or, at most, *occasional* fibrillation and increased insertional activity in a few muscles (late and minor)
5. Absence of compressive lesions of cervical spine or foramen magnum (spinal MRI scanning)
6. Absence of high signals on MRI similar to those seen in MS

Additionally suggestive of PLS
1. Preserved bladder function
2. Absent or very prolonged latency on cortical motor evoked response in the presence of normal peripheral stimulus-evoked compound muscle action potentials
3. Focal atrophy of the precentral gyrus on MRI
4. Decreased glucose consumption in pericentral region on PET scan

motor neuron features develop the diagnosis would be changed to ALS, implying that the two syndromes form a continuum or, at least, are closely related (Swash et al., 1999). There is atrophy of the precentral gyrus on MRI. The Central motor conduction time is increased, even two or three times normal (Kuipers-Upmeijer et al., 2001) in contrast to ALS in which it is usually normal. Somatosensory evoked potentials may also be of increased latency, or absent, in some patients with PLS (Kuipers-Upmeijer et al., 2001).

Familial ALS

About 5–10% of ALS/MND cases are inherited as an autosomal dominant trait (familial ALS or FALS). FALS and sporadic ALS are clinically and pathologically similar. A locus for familial ALS was reported on the long arm of chromosome 21 (Siddique et al., 1991). About 20% of FALS families have a mutation in the gene for Cu/Zn superoxide dismutase (*SOD1*). SOD enzyme activity was reduced to around 50% of normal in individuals with *SOD1* mutations (Rosen et al., 1993).

In one series, a predilection for disease onset in the lower limbs appeared to be a distinguishing feature of familial ALS with *SOD1* mutations (Orrell et al., 1997). The belief that sensory pathways are more often involved in familial ALS, arises from postmortem studies demonstrating degeneration in the posterior and Clark's columns (Hirano et al., 1967a; Hawkes et al., 1984). However, a review of familial ALS with different mutations in the *SOD1* gene, suggested that the variability of clinical phenotype associated with specific mutations in this gene is marked (Radunovic and Leigh, 1996). Distinct mutations in the *Cu/ZnSOD-1* gene are associated with a rapidly progressive form, a classic form, and a relatively benign form of ALS. However, it is thought that the phenotype of subjects with *Cu/Zn SOD1* mutations is determined by factors other than the site of the mutation. These factors could be environmental, genetic, or both (Williams et al., 1988). Caution is therefore needed in making genotype/phenotype correlations and population based studies are necessary to understand the complex gene–gene and gene–environment interactions. Andersen (2001) has reviewed the concept that sporadic ALS may have a genetic component, by considering the possibility that sporadic cases of the disease may consist of families with mutations of low penetrance.

Diagnosis of ALS

The clinical features of MND depend on the subtype of the disorder as well as the stage of the disease at which the clinical assessment is performed. In order to ensure uniformity of patient cohorts enrolled into clinical trials for assessment of potential therapies in ALS, the World Federation of Neurology proposed diagnostic clinical criteria, known as the '*El Escorial*' criteria (WFN Research Group on Neuromuscular Diseases and Subcommittee on MND/ALS, 1994).

At a meeting held in Airlie House, Virginia, these criteria were revisited (*WFN El Escorial/Airlie Criteria 1998*), and a consensus document detailing amendments to the original criteria placed on the WFN ALS website (http://www.wfnals.org/). The diagnosis of ALS now requires the **presence** of:

1 evidence of lower motor neuron (LMN) degeneration by clinical, electrophysiological or neuropathological examination,
2 evidence of upper motor neuron (UMN) degeneration by clinical examination,
3 progressive spread of symptoms or signs within a region or to other regions, as determined by history or examination.

And the **absence** of:

1 electrophysiological and pathological evidence of other disease processes that might explain the signs of LMN or UMN degeneration, and
2 neuroimaging evidence of other disease processes that might explain the observed clinical and electrophysiological signs.

Clinically definite ALS

Defined by evidence on clinical grounds alone of:

- the presence of UMN as well as LMN signs in the bulbar region and at least two spinal regions, or
- the presence of UMN signs in two spinal regions and LMN signs in three spinal regions.

Clinically probable ALS

Defined by evidence on clinical grounds alone of:

- UMN and LMN signs in at least two regions with some UMN signs rostral to (above) the LMN signs.

Probable ALS-Laboratory supported

Defined as:

- clinical evidence of UMN and LMN signs in only one region, or UMN signs alone in one region and LMN signs defined by EMG criteria in at least two limbs,

but only when proper application of neuroimaging and clinical laboratory protocols has excluded other causes.

Possible ALS

Defined by evidence of:

▓ UMN and LMN signs in only one region, or
▓ UMN signs alone in two or more regions, or
▓ LMN signs found rostral to UMN signs.

Other diagnoses must have been excluded.

Traditionally, the diagnosis of ALS has been substantiated by electrophysiological studies utilizing criteria formulated by Lambert and Mulder (1957). These were subsequently modified by the exclusion of patients with motor conduction block (Cornblath et al., 1992) and recently confirmed by consensus at Airlie House, Virginia (Table 1.5). These EMG signs of LMN dysfunction should be found in at least two of the four body regions: bulbar/cranial, cervical, thoracic, and lumbosacral.

Table 1.5 Electrophysiological evidence in the diagnosis of ALS (Airlie House criteria 1998)

Signs of active denervation
• fibrillation potentials
• Positive sharp waves

Fasciculations

Signs of chronic partial denervation
• Motor unit potentials of increased duration and amplitude with high proportion of polyphasia
• Reduced interference pattern, usually with high firing rates, e.g. higher than 10Hz
• Unstable motor unit potentials
• Chronic partial denervation could also be demonstrated by other techniques, e.g. SFEMG, macro-EMG, turns-amplitude analysis, quantitative MUP analysis, and MUNE

Features compatible with UMN involvement
• Up to 30% increase in central motor conduction time
• Low firing rates of motor unit potentials on effort

Features suggesting other disease processes
• Evidence of motor conduction block
• Motor conduction velocity lower than 70% of lower limit of normal
• Distal motor latency greater than 30% above upper limit of normal
• Abnormal sensory nerve conduction studies except in the presence of entrapment syndromes or coexisting peripheral nerve disease
• F-wave or H-reflex latencies more than 30% above established normal values
• Decrements greater than 20% on repetitive stimulation
• SSEP latency greater than 20% of established normal value
• Significant abnormalities in autonomic function or electronystagmography
• Full motor unit potential interference pattern in a clinically weak muscle

Geographic and ethnic variations in the clinical presentation of motor neuron diseases

The description of motor neuron diseases from different parts of the world differs from classical ALS in many aspects. Some of these conditions are described below (Table 1.6).

Ben Hamida et al. (1990) described from Tunisia an unusual form of autosomal recessive, childhood onset motor neuron disease characterized by chronic

Table 1.6 Geographic variants of ALS/MND

- Juvenile ALS – Tunisia
- Madras motor neuron disease
- Monomelic amyotrophy/wasted leg syndrome
- Lathyrism
- Konzo
- ALS parkinsonism dementia complex of Guam

slowly progressive degeneration of both upper and lower motor neurons. The anatomical distribution of clinical features is identical to that in classical ALS. A combination of upper and lower motor neuron dysfunction often associated with pseudobulbar changes is characteristic of this form of 'juvenile ALS'. Cognitive and sensory function remain intact, and survival over several decades is the rule. Genetic linkage of a large pedigree with juvenile ALS has defined a disease locus on the distal long arm of chromosome 2 (Hentati et al., 1994).

'Madras motor neuron disease' is the term applied to a sporadic, slowly progressive, juvenile onset of asymmetric weakness and wasting of the limbs accompanied by bulbar dysfunction, bilateral facial involvement, and deafness (Meenakshisundaram et al., 1970). The presence of UMN signs is variable, and the clinical course is benign. Survival over several decades is frequent. The etiology of this condition is obscure.

'Monomelic amyotrophy' is a condition characterized by weakness and wasting limited to the fingers, hand, forearm and occasionally arm of a single limb in young persons aged 15–25 years (Singh et al., 1980; Hirayama et al., 1987). The abnormality may progress mildly to involve the opposite limb over 1–4 years and then the disorder arrests or advances minimally with little functional disability. Fasciculations are observed, UMN signs are absent, while sensation and sphincters are normal. Occasional familial cases of this benign disorder occurring in Japan, India, and China suggest either recessive or dominant inheritance.

'Lathyrism', described from India (Ludolph et al., 1987), and 'Konzo', described from Central Africa (Tylleskar et al., 1993), are pure UMN syndromes having abrupt onset of nonprogressive weakness in the lower limbs. There is no LMN involvement. They have been linked to the consumption of chickling pea and cassava roots, respectively, in drought prone lands, with resultant neurotoxicity from BOAA (beta-oxalyl-amino-alanine) and dietary cyanide.

Compared with classic ALS, the profile of **ALS in Guam,** the Kii Peninsula of Japan, and West New Guinea shows certain differences (Hirano et al., 1967b). It is typically a disease of early onset, of longer duration, and associated with an increased frequency of parkinsonism and dementia. Clinical and neuropathological studies suggest that there are two syndromes, one with an ALS-like presentation, and another in which there is a parkinsonism/dementia complex (McGeer et al., 1997). There is continuing debate as to the role of genetic and environmental factors in the etiology of these syndromes.

Disorders that could be mistaken for ALS

Before making a diagnosis of ALS, it is vital to ensure that 'mimic syndromes' that may masquerade as ALS have been ruled out since these have different

Table 1.7 Disorders that may resemble ALS

- SMAs – adult-onset proximal SMA, Kennedy's syndrome
- Physical injury – radiation myelopathy, post-traumatic syringomyelia
- Endocrine diseases – thyrotoxicosis and hyperparathyroidism
- Immune mediated – paraproteinemic and multifocal motor neuropathies
- Exogenous toxins – lead and mercury
- Tumors – lymphoma and cancer associated neuromuscular syndromes
- Inherited enzyme defects – hexosaminidase deficiency
- Sjögren's syndrome
- Postinfectious – postpolio amyotrophy

prognoses, and some are treatable. The following conditions should be considered in the differential diagnosis of ALS (Table 1.7).

Spinal muscular atrophy

Adult onset proximal SMA may mimic progressive muscular atrophy in its presentation with an asymmetric, limb restricted weakness and wasting, without UMN signs (Serratrice, 1983). Bulbar muscles are rarely affected. SMA is usually proximal but distal onset SMA syndromes are recognized (Pearn and Hudgson, 1979). SMAs of late onset progress only slowly, and survival is much longer than in classic MND. Autosomal recessive inheritance may be observed in familial cases, though sporadic cases are more common. It is often difficult to distinguish sporadic adult-onset proximal SMA from PMA. The clinical features of the two can be identical, except for a more rapid rate of progress in progressive muscular atrophy. Most SMA syndromes are linked to a mutation on chromosome 5q. 13 (Melki, 1997).

Kennedy's syndrome

Kennedy's syndrome (bulbospinal neuronopathy) is an X-linked recessive disorder, characterized by the onset of weakness and wasting in the girdle muscles in men aged 40–50 years (Kennedy et al., 1968). The tongue is almost always involved eventually. It is preceded by the presence of arm tremors, muscle cramps and generalized fasciculations in the previous 10–15 years. Perioral fasciculations, wasting of the tongue, and bulbar dysfunction develop. Gynecomastia, testicular atrophy with azoospermia and diabetes are noted in some patients. The progress of the disease is slow, and disability is not severe. Neurophysiological evaluation reveals reduced or absent sensory nerve action potentials besides widespread chronic partial denervation with evidence of reinnervation on EMG. A mutation in the coding region of the androgen receptor gene results in variable increase in the number of CAG tandem repeats at this site (LaSpada et al., 1991). This can be detected by a PCR test performed on peripheral blood leukocyte DNA.

Radiation myelopathy

A LMN syndrome has been reported 3 months to 13 years after radiation to the para-aortic spinal region for malignant testicular and lymphomatous tumors (Bradley et al., 1991). The syndrome occurred when the radiation dosage exceeded 4000 rad. Asymmetric weakness, atrophy, fasciculations, cramps and areflexia were cardinal features. Sensory, sphincter, and pyramidal tract involvement were not observed. The clinical abnormalities progressed over 1–2 years before stabilizing. Magnetic resonance imaging studies of the spinal cord were normal. Sensory and motor nerve conduction studies were normal, as were somatosensory evoked responses. Needle EMG showed evidence of chronic partial denervation with reinnervation in affected and some clinically unaffected muscles. This syndrome resulted from an endothelial vasculopathy of the spinal cord leading to anterior horn cell degeneration. There is an extensive older literature related to radiation therapy for lung, breast, oral, and maxillofacial cancer, but the syndrome is rare in modern oncologic practice.

Endocrine dysfunction

ALS-like syndromes have been described in patients with thyrotoxicosis. Separating these syndromes from classical ALS can be difficult as both may exhibit diffuse fasciculations, muscle wasting, weight loss, brisk reflexes and even bulbar dysfunction. The syndrome may result from a combination of myelopathy, myopathy and motor neuropathy due to thyrotoxicosis, as resolution of the symptoms and signs follows treatment of the thyroid disorder (Fisher et al., 1985). The presence of exophthalmos and postural tremor of the outstretched hands are useful clinical clues to the underlying condition. The diagnosis is established by performing thyroid function tests.

80% of patients with primary hyperparathyrodism, 60% of patients with secondary hyperparathyroidism, and patients with hypophosphatemic osteomalacia develop pelvifemoral weakness and wasting. Bone pain is characteristically present but the presence of fasciculations, hyperreflexia and Babinski signs may cause confusion with ALS (Patten and Engel, 1982). The EMG may show predominantly neurogenic features, but myopathic features may also be present, especially in osteomalacia (Pattern and Engel, 1982; Dubas et al., 1989; Trebini et al., 1993). Treatment of hypophosphatemia with oral phosphate replacement and removal of adenomatous parathyroids results in reversal of this ALS-like disorder.

Multifocal motor neuropathy

Multifocal motor neuropathy (MMN) can closely mimic ALS. The clinical hallmarks of MMN are the onset of slowly progressive asymmetric weakness and wasting presenting between the third and fifth decade. The distribution of affected muscles is often confined to the territory of individual nerves, which with multiple nerve involvement may mimic global limb weakness. The upper limbs are first and often more severely affected (Bouche et al., 1995). Marked weakness in occasional muscles without significant wasting, and depression of tendon reflexes, are clinical clues to the diagnosis. However, in some cases the separation of MMN from classical ALS may be blurred due to the presence of brisk reflexes, muscle cramps, and diffuse fasciculations in MMN (Pestronk et al., 1990). Rarely, involvement of the tongue makes the similarity to ALS complete (Kaji et al., 1992). However, the rate of progression is slower in MMN than in ALS. Nerve conduction studies in MMN reveal the conduction block (CB) or partial conduction block (PCB), a *sine qua non* for the diagnosis. Although Pestronk et al. (1990) stressed the finding of increased titers of anti-GM1 ganglioside IgM antibodies in 77% of their 25 cases, subsequent studies have lessened the value of this test as a marker of this disorder. A favorable response to intravenous cyclophosphamide therapy (Feldman et al., 1991) and immunoglobulin injections (Chaudhry et al., 1993) has been noted in varying degrees. The long-term response to these treatments is unknown.

There have been only three pathological studies of MMN at autopsy (Adams et al., 1993; Oh et al., 1995; Veugelers et al., 1996). Two of these reported the presence of demyelination and axonal loss in the anterior spinal roots associated with loss of anterior horn cells in the ventral spinal cord (Adams et al., 1993; Oh et al., 1995). In the third report, characteristic clinical features of MMN were noted, but the patient failed to respond to intravenous cyclophosphamide therapy and died after 19 months of illness (Veugelers et al., 1996). The autopsy revealed patchy areas of demyelination underlying areas of recorded conduction block on NCV studies, but there was loss of anterior horn cells and axonal loss in the corticospinal tracts, features consistent (as in the other two autopsies) with ALS. This has raised doubts about the status of MMN as a unique disease entity, and about the diagnostic criteria for MMN.

Toxic exposure
Lead

Acute intoxication due to lead produces an encephalopathy in children and adults, whereas chronic exposure leads to behavioral disturbances and a motor neuropathy. Heavy and prolonged exposure to lead has also been associated with a motor disorder characterized by marked weakness and atrophy beginning in the arms, with fasciculations, bulbar dysfunction, hyperreflexia, spasticity, and Babinski signs (Conradi et al., 1982; Adams et al., 1983). Only a history of exposure to lead, rather slow progression of events, and a response to chelation therapy can differentiate this disorder from classic ALS. Anorexia, abdominal pain, constipation and a blue leadline in the gums may be clues to the diagnosis. Laboratory features include anemia, basophilic stippling of RBCs, and increased blood and urinary lead levels.

Mercury

Workers involved in the manufacture of electrical equipment, paint, paper, pulp, cosmetics, and nuclear devices may suffer from accidental mercury intoxication. This produces myalgia, weight loss, irritability, photophobia, abdominal pain, tremors, behavioral changes and ataxia (Mitchell, 1987). Rarely, brief but significant exposure to mercury may produce a rapid development of an ALS-like disorder with muscle atrophy, fasciculations, and hyperreflexia (Barber, 1978). The rapid evolution and the presence of other systemic symptoms with swollen gums and blue lines are indicative of the disorder.

Paraneoplastic disorders

An ALS-like syndrome was reported in 9 cases over a 10 year period, in conjunction with Hodgkin's and non-Hodgkin's lymphoma, and chronic lymphocytic leukemia (Younger et al., 1991). Asymmetric LMN involvement with a predilection for males was observed. Additional UMN signs and sensory abnormalities were noted in some. The relationship among ALS, lymphoproliferative disease, and the presence of paraproteinemia on serum immunoelectrophoresis has been discussed most extensively by Gordon et al. (1997). They suggest that an elevated CSF protein may signal the presence of underlying lymphoproliferative disease in patients with MND in whom investigations reveal a monoclonal gammopathy and a raised ESR. In one of their patients with clinical features of ALS, in whom investigations revealed the presence of a paraprotein and elevated ESR, underlying disseminated lymphoma was detected only at autopsy. In another study, low-level IgM antibodies to gangliosides GM1 and GD1a were detected in a proportion of patients with ALS without underlying lymphoproliferative disease (Pestronk et al., 1989). The authors hypothesized that autoimmune mechanisms may be involved in the pathogenesis of some cases of ALS (Drachman and Kuncl, 1989). It is possible that ALS-like syndromes associated with lymphoproliferative diseases are immune mediated.

Clinical features typical of PLS and ALS have also been reported in association with carcinoma of the breast and oat cell carcinoma of the lung respectively (Forsyth et al., 1997), suggesting that motor neuron syndromes could be included in the list of paraneoplastic disorders (Rowland, 1997). Clinically, underlying cancer may be suspected in a patient with onset of a motor neuron disorder before 30 and after 70 years of age, showing an acute or subacute progression. The presence of subtle sensory dysfunction, and a pure LMN or pure UMN syndrome should deepen the suspicion. Thus in patients with apparent ALS, an atypically rapid course, a 'pure' syndrome, the presence of a paraprotein, elevated CSF protein, or an elevated ESR on investigation should prompt a search for underlying neoplasm.

Postpolio syndrome (postpolio amyotrophy)

'Postpolio amyotrophy' is the term applied to new onset of muscle weakness and fatigue decades after recovery from acute poliomyelitis. Progressive weakness, atrophy, and fasciculation simulates motor neuron disease (Dalakas et al., 1986). The previous history of poliomyelitis, absence of UMN signs, slow rate of progression, the presence of pain without demonstrable cause, and occurrence of new amyotrophy at the border zone of prior paralysis where regeneration might predominate should all raise the suspicion of postpolio amyotrophy.

Hexosaminidase deficiency

An ALS-like syndrome may be inherited in an autosomal recessive manner in patients of Ashkenazi Jewish descent. A combination of upper and lower motor neuron dysfunction in the third to fifth decade is associated with the variable presence of ataxia, stuttering, dementia, psychosis or polyneuropathy. In some instances a family history of Tay-Sachs disease is obtained. The disorder is caused by a genetic absence of the lysosomal hydrolase enzyme N-acetyl-β hexosaminidase A, the activity of which can be measured in the serum, leukocytes, and cultured fibroblasts (Mitsumoto et al., 1985). The finding of low activity of this enzyme in patients and in asymptomatic relatives is of relevance for establishing the diagnosis and for genetic counselling.

Autoimmune disorders

An ALS- and PLS-like syndrome has been described in patients with primary Sjögren's syndrome (Salachas et al., 1998). Some of these patients stabilized or improved after institution of corticosteroid therapy. The mechanisms underlying the neurological manifestations are unknown.

Investigations when ALS is suspected

A detailed history and meticulous neurologic assessment lay the foundation for relevant investigations in a patient with suspected ALS. Vigilance for the presence of atypical features e.g. mode of onset, age, rate of progression, presence of associated systemic or other neurological features, and the presence of 'pure syndromes' assist the recognition of ALS-mimic syndromes. Every patient with suspected ALS should undergo baseline liver function tests, as these may be altered by riluzole, currently the standard therapy for ALS. Hematological studies, including an ESR, are mandatory, as lymphoproliferative disorders masquerading as motor neuron disease may be unmasked by abnormal results of these investigations. Elevated protein or an abnormal cell count in the CSF suggest causes other than ALS.

MRI scanning of the brain and spinal cord is usually normal in ALS except for the detection of occasional T2-weighted hyperintensities in the course of the corticospinal tracts, and atrophy of the precentral gyrus on use of high strength magnetic coils. Abnormal results on MR imaging help in excluding conditions mimicking ALS in the early stages (see Chapter 2).

Sensory and motor nerve conduction studies are usually normal in ALS, except for decrease in amplitudes of distal CMAPs. Concentric needle EMG reveals changes of chronic partial denervation with reinnervation in a widespread distribution, accompanied by diffuse fasciculations. The motor unit potentials (MUPs) are reduced in number and of increased amplitude and duration. On maximal voluntary activation the recruitment pattern is reduced. The distribution of these changes has to be beyond the anatomical territories of peripheral nerves and nerve roots for the diagnosis of ALS to be corroborated. At least two proximal and two distal muscles in all four limbs should be sampled on concentric needle EMG. The presence of fasciculations at rest in the tongue, either clinically or on EMG, has a high specificity for the diagnosis of ALS, especially when other clinical features are consistent.

The presence of prolonged F-wave responses, dispersion of CMAPs, conduction block, and slowing of motor conduction velocities are hallmarks of multifocal motor neuropathy. The presence of sensory dysfunction on sensory nerve conduction studies differentiates Kennedy's syndrome from motor neuron disease.

Additional investigations may be performed on the basis of the algorithm shown in Figure 1.1.

Early diagnosis

The revised '*El Escorial*' criteria (World Federation of Neurology, 1994; Airlie House revision, 1998) are useful in the diagnosis of the classic syndrome. However, by definition a patient would have fairly advanced biological disease at the time of diagnosis. Early in the illness, focal weakness and/or atrophy, nonspecific symptoms like fatigue, weight loss, and fasciculations may occur. At this stage, the disorder is often mistaken for lumbar or cervical radiculopathy, compression palsy of a peripheral nerve, or brachial or lumbosacral plexus lesion, etc. At this early stage, no specific biological test or investigation is available to establish the diagnosis. There is an imperative need to develop a test or criteria for the early diagnosis of ALS. The measurement of 'threshold electro-tonus' failed to sustain the initial promise as one such investigative technique (Bostock et al., 1995). Early diagnosis is increasingly important in the current era of emerging treatments.

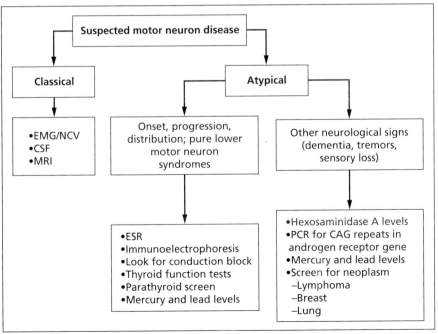

Fig. 1.1 Algorithm for investigative approach to a patient with suspected motor neuron disease

ALS: principles of management

ALS is a progressive disorder that invariably results in death. Having made the diagnosis, the treating physician must convey the news truthfully to the patient and then help them cope with disability, the prospect of death, and the accompanying human fears and frustrations. Good communication skills, honesty and empathy for the patient's plight pave the way for a balanced relationship between patient and physician. Symptomatic management includes the use of antispasticity agents, anticramping agents, antidepressants, drying agents for sialorrhea, respiratory agents, and vaccines against influenza and pneumococcus. A multidisciplinary approach has to be formulated to plan nutritional management and physical rehabilitation (see Chapter 7). Though numerous potential therapies have been tested in extensive and expensive trials, none has found to have a curative effect (reviewed in detail in Chapter 8).

In two large, randomized, double-blind, placebo-controlled trials, the antiglutamate agent riluzole has been shown to improve tracheostomy-free survival when compared with placebo (Bensimon et al., 1994; Lacomblez et al., 1996). A Cox proportional hazards analysis was used to adjust for bad prognostic features such as bulbar onset, reduced vital capacity, rapid progression, and advanced disease (Wagner and Landis, 1997). This has generated enthusiasm and support in pursuing research in quest of a cure for this disorder. However, conducting clinical trials for putative treatments for ALS is fraught with numerous difficulties and dilemmas that require further consideration (discussed in Chapters 8 and 9). The major current clinical problem is early diagnosis.

References

Abrahams S, Goldstein LH, Kew JJM et al. (1996) Frontal lobe dysfunction in amyotrophic lateral sclerosis. A PET study. Brain 119: 2105–2120.

Abrahams S, Goldstein LH, Al-Chalabi A et al. (1997) Relation between cognitive dysfunction and pseudobulbar palsy in amyotrophic lateral sclerosis. J Neurol Neurosurg Psychiatry 62(5): 464–472.

Adams CR, Zeigler DK, Lin JT (1983) Mercury intoxication simulating amyotrophic lateral sclerosis. JAMA 250: 642–643.

Adams D, Kuntzer T, Steck AJ, Lobrinus A, Janzer RC, Regli F (1993) Motor conduction block and high titres of anti-GM1 ganglioside antibodies: pathological evidence of a motor neuropathy in a patient with lower motor neuron syndrome. J Neurol Neurosurg Psychiatry 56: 982–987.

Andersen PM. Genetics of sporadic ALS. ALS 2001; 2 (Suppl.1): S37–S41.

Aran FA (1850) Recherches sur une maladie non encore décrite du système musculaire (Atrophie musculaire progressive). Arch Gen Med 24: 5–35, 172–214.

Barber TE (1978) Inorganic mercury poisoning reminiscent of amyotrophic lateral sclerosis. J Occup Med 20: 667–669.

Beasley WC (1961) Quantitative muscle testing: principles and application to research and clinical services. Arch Phys Med Rehabil 42: 398–425.

Ben Hamida M, Hentati F, Ben Hamida C (1990) Hereditary motor system diseases (chronic juvenile amyotrophic lateral sclerosis). Brain 113: 347–363.

Bensimon G, Lacomblez L, Meininger V, ALS/Riluzole Study Group (1994) A controlled trial of riluzole in amyotrophic lateral sclerosis. N Engl J Med 330: 585–591.

Bostock H, Sharief MK, Reid MG, Murray NMF (1995) Axonal ion channel dysfunction in amyotrophic lateral sclerosis. Brain 118: 217–225.

Bouche P, Moulonguet A, Younes-Chennoufi AB et al. (1995) Multifocal motor neuropathy with conduction block: a study of 24 patients. J Neurol Neurosurg Psychiatry 59: 38–44.

Bradley WG, Robison SH, Tandan R, Besser D (1991) Post-radiation motor neuron syndromes. Adv Neurol 56: 341–353.

Brain WR (1962) In: Diseases of the nervous system, 6th Ed. Oxford University Press: Oxford, pp 531.

Chaudhry V, Corse AM, Cornblath DR et al. (1993) Multifocal motor neuropathy: response to human immune globulin. Ann Neurol 33: 237–242.

Charcot JM, Joffroy A (1869) Deux cas d'atrophie musculaire progressive avec lésions de la substance grise et des faisceaux antéro-latéraux de la moelle épinière. Arch Physiol Neurol Path 2: 744.

Conradi S, Ronnevi LO, Norris FH (1982) Motor neuron disease and toxic metals. Adv Neurol 36: 201–231.

Cornblath DR, Kuncl RW, Mellits D et al. (1992) Nerve conduction studies in amyotrophic lateral sclerosis. Muscle Nerve 15: 1111–1115.

Cruveilhier J (1852–1853) Sur la paralysie musculaire, progressive, atrophique. Bull Acad Med (Paris) 18: 490–546.

Dalakas MC, Elder G, Hallet M (1986) A long-term follow-up study of patients with postpoliomyelitis neuromuscular symptoms. N Eng J Med 314: 959–963.

Drachman DB, Kuncl RW (1989) Amyotrophic lateral sclerosis: an unconventional autoimmune disease? Ann Neurol 26(2): 269–274.

Dubas F, Bertrand P, Emile J (1989) Progressive spinal muscular atrophy and parathyroid adenoma. Clinico-pahological study of a case. Rev Neurol 145: 65–68.

Duchenne de Boulogne GBA (1849) Recherches faites à l'orde des galvanisine sur l'état de la contractilité et de la sensibilité électromusculaires dans les paralysies des membres supérieurs. CR Acad Sci (Paris) 29: 667.

Duchenne de Boulogne GBA (1860) Paralysie musculaire progressive de la langue, du voile du palais et des lèvres: affection non encore décrite comme espèce morbide distincte. Arch Gén Méd 16: 283, 431.

Erb WH (1891) Dystrophie muscularis progressiva: Klinische und pathologisch-anatomische studien. Dtsch Nervenheilk 1: 13–94, 173–261.

Feldman EL, Bromberg MB, Albers JW et al. (1991) Immunosuppressive treatment in multifocal motor neuropathy. Ann Neurol 30: 397–401.

Fisher M, Mateer JE, Ullrich I, Gutrecht JA (1985) Pyramidal tact deficits and polyneuropathy in hyperthyroidism: combination clinically mimicking amyotrophic lateral sclerosis. Am J Med 78: 1041–1044.

Forsyth PA, Dalmau J, Graus F, Cwik V, Rosenblum MK, Posner JB (1997) Motor neuron syndromes in cancer patients. Ann Neurol 41: 722–730.

Gordon PH, Rowland LP, Younger DS et al. (1997) Lymphoproliferative disorders and motor neuron disease: an update. Neurology 48: 1671–1678.

Hawkes CH, Cavanaugh JB, Mowbray S, Paul EA (1984) Familial motor neurone disease: report of a family with five post-morterm studies. In: Rose FE (Ed.) Research Progress in Motor Neurone Disease. Pitman: London, pp. 70–78.

Hentati A, Bejaoui K, Pericak-Vance MA et al. (1994) Linkage of recessive familial amyotrophic lateral sclerosis to chromosome 2q33-35. Nature Genetics 7: 425–428.

Hirano A, Kurland LT, Sayre GP (1967a) Familial amyotrophic lateral sclerosis: a subgroup characterised by posterior and spinocerebellar tract involvement and hyaline inclusions in the anterior horn cells. Arch Neurol 16: 232–243.

Hirano A, Arumugasamy N, Zimmerman HM (1967b) Amyotrophic lateral sclerosis: a comparison of Guam and classic cases. Arch Neurol 16: 357–363.

Hirayama K, Tomonaga M, Kitano K, Yamada T, Kojima S, Arai K (1987) Focal cervical poliopathy causing juvenile muscular atrophy of distal upper extremity: a pathological study. J Neurol Neurosurg Psychiatry 50: 285–290.

Jablecki CK, Berry C, Leach J (1989) Survival prediction in amyotrophic lateral sclerosis. Muscle Nerve 12: 833–841.

Jackson M, Lennox G, Lowe J (1996) Motor neuron disease-inclusion dementia. Neurodegeneration 5: 339–350.

Kaji R, Shibasaki H, Kimura J (1992) Multifocal motor neuropathy: cranial nerve involvement and immunoglobulin therapy. Neurology 42: 506–509.

Kennedy WR, Alter M, Sung JH (1968) Progressive proximal spinal and bulbar muscular atrophy of late onset: a sex-linked recessive trait. Neurology 18: 671–680.

Kuipers-Upmeijer J, de Jager AEJ, Snock JW, van Weerden TW. Primary lateral sclerosis: clinical, neurophysiological and magnetic resonance findings. J Neurol Neurosurg Phychiatry 2001; 71: 615–620.

Lacomblez L, Bensimon G, Leigh PN, ALS/Riluzole Study Group II (1996) Dose-ranging study of riluzole in amyotrophic lateral sclerosis. Lancet 347: 1425–1431.

Lambert EH, Mulder DW (1957) Electromyographic studies in amyotrophic lateral sclerosis. Proc Mayo Clinic Staff 32: 427–436.

LaSpada AR, Wilson EM, Lubahn DB, Harding AE, Fischbeck KH (1991) Androgen receptor gene mutations in X-linked spinal and bulbar muscular atrophy. Nature 352: 77–79.

Lawyer T, Netsky MG (1953) Amyotrophic lateral sclerosis: a clinico-anatomic study of fifty-three cases. Arch Neurol Psychiat 69: 171–192.

Ludolph AC, Hugon J, Dwivedi MP, Schaumberg HH, Spencer PS (1987) Studies on the aetiology and pathogenesis of motor neuron diseases: 1. Lathyrism: clinical findings in established cases. Brain 110: 149–165.

Luys JB (1860) Atrophie musculaire progressive. Lésions histologiques de la substance grise de la moelle épinière. Gaz Med (Paris) 15: 505.

McComas AJ (1991) Invited Review. Motor unit estimation: Methods, results and present status. Muscle Nerve 14: 585–597.

McGeer PL, Schwab C, McGeer EG, Haddock RL, Steele JC (1997) Familial nature and continuing morbidity of the amyotrophic lateral sclerosis-parkinsonism dementia complex of Guam. Neurology 49: 400–409.

Meenakshisundaram E, Jaggannathan K, Ramamurthi B (1970) Clinical pattern of motor neuron disease seen in younger age groups in Madras. Neurol India 18: 109.

Melki J (1997) Spinal muscular atrophy. Curr Opin Neurol 10(5): 381–385.

Mitchell JD (1987) Heavy metals and trace elements in amyotrophic lateral sclerosis. Neurol Clin 5: 43–60.

Mitsumoto H, Sliman RJ, Schafer IA et al. (1985) Motor neuron disease and adult hexosaminidase deficiency in two families: evidence for multisystem degeneration. Ann Neurol 17: 378–385.

Mulder DW, Howard FM (1976) Patient resistance and prognosis in amyotrophic lateral sclerosis. Mayo Clin Proc 51: 537–541.

Neary D, Snowden JS, Mann DMA et al. (1990) Frontal lobe dementia and motor neuron disease. J Neurol Neurosurg Psychiatry 53: 23–32.

Oh SJ, Claussen GC, Odabasi Z, Palmer CP (1995) Multifocal demyelinating motor neuropathy: pathologic evidence of 'inflammatory demyelinating polyradiculoneuropathy'. Neurology 45: 1828–1832.

Orrell RW, Habgood JJ, Gardiner I et al. (1997) Clinical and functional investigation of 10 missense mutations and a novel frameshift insertion mutation of the gene for copper-zinc superoxide dismutase in UK families with amyotrophic lateral sclerosis. Neurology 48(3): 746–751.

Parry GJ, Sumner AJ (1992) Multifocal motor neuropathy. Neurol Clin 10: 671–684.

Pattern BM, Engel WK (1982) Phosphate and parathyroid disorders associated with the syndrome of amyotrophic lateral sclerosis. Adv Neurol 36: 181–200.

Pearn J, Hudgson P (1979) Distal spinal muscular atrophy. A clinical and genetic study of 8 kindreds. J Neurol Sci 43: 183–191.

Pestronk A, Adams RN, Cornblath DR, Kuncl RW, Drachman DB, Clawson L (1989) Patterns of serum IgM antibodies to GM1 and GD1a gangliosides in amyotrophic lateral sclerosis. Ann Neurol 25(1): 98–102.

Pestronk A, Chaudhry V, Feldman EL et al. (1990) Lower motor neuron syndromes defined by patterns of weakness, nerve conduction abnormalities, and high titres of antiglycolipid antibodies. Ann Neurol 27: 316–326.

Pringle CE, Hudson AJ, Munoz DG, Kiernan JA, Brown WF, Ebers GC (1992) Primary lateral sclerosis: clinical features, neuropathology and diagnostic criteria. Brain 115: 495–520.

Qureshi AI, Wilmot G, Dihenia B, Schneider JA, Krendel DA (1996) Motor neuron disease with parkinsonism. Arch Neurol 53: 987–991.

Radunovic A, Leigh PN on behalf of the European Familial ALS Group (1996) Cu/Zn superoxide dismutase gene mutations in amyotrophic lateral sclerosis: correlation between genotype and clinical features. J Neurol Neurosurg Psychiatry 61: 565–572.

Rosen DR, Siddique T, Patterson D et al. (1993) Mutations in Cu/Zn superoxide dismutase gene are associated with familial amyotrophic lateral sclerosis. Nature 362: 59–62.

Rowland LP (1982) Diverse forms of motor neuron disease. In: Rowland LP (Ed) Human Motor Neuron Diseases. Raven Press: New York, pp. 1–13.

Rowland LP (1997) Paraneoplastic primary lateral sclerosis and amyotrophic lateral sclerosis. Ann Neurol 41: 703–705.

Salachas F, Lafitte C, Chassande B et al. (1998) Motor neuron disease mimicking amyotrophic lateral sclerosis and primary lateral sclerosis in primary Sjögren's syndrome (abstract). Neurology 50 (Suppl 4): A31.

Serratrice G (1983) Classification of adult onset chronic spinal muscular atrophies. Cardiomyology 2: 255–276.

Siddique T, Figlewicz DA, Pericak-Vance MA et al. (1991) Linkage of a gene causing familial amyotrophic lateral sclerosis to chromosome 21 and evidence of locus heterogeneity. N Engl J Med 324: 1381–1384.

Singh N, Sachdev KK, Susheela AK (1980) Juvenile muscular atrophy localised to arms. Arch Neurol 37: 297–299.

Spiller WG (1904) Primary degeneration of the pyramidal tracts: a study of eight cases with necropsy. Univ PA Med Bull 17: 390–395.

Swash M, Desai J, Misra VP. what is primary lateral sclerosis? J Neurol Sci 1999; 170:5–10.

Swash M, Ingram D (1988) Preclinical and subclinical events in motor neuron disease. J Neurol Neurosurg Psychiatry 51: 165–168.

Swash M, Leader M, Brown A, Swettenham KW (1986) Focal loss of anterior horn cells in the cervical cord in motor neuron disease. Brain 109: 939–952.

Swash M, Scholtz CL, Vowles G, Ingram DA (1988) Selective and asymmetric vulnerability of corticospinal and spinocerebellar tracts in motor neuron disease. J Neurol Neurosurg Psychiatry 51: 785–789.

Tan YD, Dolan P, Brooks BR (1988) Symptom progression in amyotrophic lateral sclerosis. Ann Neurol 24: 14A.

Trebini F, Appioti A, Bacci R, Daniele D, Inglezis A (1993) Neurological complications in hyperparathyroidism. Minerva Med 84: 73–75.

Tylleskar T, Howlett WP, Rwiza HT et al. (1993) Konzo: a distinct disease entity with selective upper motor neuron damage. J Neurol Neurosurg Psychiatry 56: 638–645.

Vejjajiva A, Foster JB, Miller H (1967) Motor neuron disease. A clinical study. J Neurol Sci 4: 299–314.

Veugelers B, Theys P, Lammens M, Van Hees J, Robberecht W (1996) Pathological findings in a patient with amyotrophic lateral sclerosis and multifocal motor neuropathy with conduction block. J Neurol Sci 136: 64–70.

Wagner ML, Landis BE (1997) Riluzole: A new agent for amyotrophic lateral sclerosis. Ann Pharmacother 31: 738–43.

Williams DB, Floate DA, Leicester J (1988) Familial motor neuron disease: differing penetrance in large pedigrees. J Neurol Sci 86: 215–230.

World Federation of Neurology Research Group on Neuromuscular Diseases and Subcommittee on Motor Neuron Diseases/Amyotrophic Lateral Sclerosis (1994) El Escorial World Federation of Neurology criteria for the diagnosis of amyotrophic lateral sclerosis. J Neurol Sci 124(Suppl): 96–107.

Younger DS, Chou S, Hays AP (1988) Primary lateral sclerosis: a clinical diagnosis re-emerges. Arch Neurol 45: 1304–1307.

Younger DS, Rowland LP, Latov N et al. (1991) Lymphoma, motor neuron diseases and amyotrophic lateral sclerosis. Ann Neurol 29: 78–86.

CHAPTER 2

Errors in diagnosis

Ralph W. Kuncl

The previous chapter provided straightforward guidelines and currently accepted international criteria for the diagnosis of motor neuron diseases. It may appear from the foregoing that the clinical diagnosis of amyotrophic lateral sclerosis, the most common motor neuron disease, is straightforward. In fact, some investigators have implied that the diagnosis is virtually always correct: in the words of a noted authority ['In our experience the clinical diagnosis of ALS is usually correct. There has been no formal assessment of this . . . but we have estimated that the diagnosis is correct in at least ninety-five percent of cases. That is, post-mortem examination confirms the diagnosis almost all the time. . . . '] (Rowland, 1997). If that is true, one need not think much about the differential diagnosis of the disease, as the course of disease will eventually declare itself. Others have argued that the rate of misdiagnosis is rather high, perhaps 15% or higher. The truth is probably somewhere in between and probably depends on the kind of referral sources that make up the cachement of the investigator, whether secondary, tertiary, or late tertiary.

Diagnostic pressure in the clinical trials era and what can be learned from erroneous diagnoses

The learning is in the errors. Thoughtful consideration of erroneous diagnoses can lead to a more analytical approach and then to diagnostic algorithms like those presented in Chapter 1 and here. Although the presentation of ALS *is* often distinctive and the diagnosis straightforward, early in the disease diagnosis is frequently difficult. This is becoming more and more of an issue in the practice of clinical trials as more clinical trials abound and as patients enter them earlier. Those conducting clinical trials well know that probably every large trial has inadvertently included patients who turned out later to have such diseases as multifocal motor neuropathy or spondylotic amyotrophy. Every seasoned clinician knows that confusing patients often include those with myelographically proven spondylosis and multilevel root disease but relentless motor progression. This issue is more than a theoretical problem, because the incidence of ALS is age related; many cases occur in the sixth to eighth decades when spondylosis and minor sensory changes are also common.

Often, a neurological examination repeated at intervals is the ultimate confirmatory test, as the combination of inexorable progression of upper and lower motor neuron signs makes the diagnosis obvious. However, the luxury of the test of time is meaningless to the patient in the current therapeutic era who wants to receive neuroprotective treatments and experimental approaches as soon as feasible. It is also a barrier to the clinical trialist who wants to enter patients in increasingly large multicenter trials. The pressure towards earlier diagnosis is real; the flow of patients into clinical trials encounters the opposite obstacle of higher rates of misdiagnosis earlier in the course of disease. Some large study groups have modified the WFN (1994; 1998) diagnostic criteria to shave a few months off the mean lag between onset and diagnosis, but the validity of such efforts is limited by short follow-up times and absence of pathological confirmation of diagnosis (Ross et al., 1998).

Prior research on the nature and rate of misdiagnosis
Case reports and case series in the literature

Numerous case reports, often presented only in abstract form, have highlighted patients with apparent ALS-like presentations who had other disorders, such as multiple nerve entrapments, multifocal motor neuropathy, carcinomas, and many other diseases, including even such unexpected mimics as Sjögren's syndrome (Salachas et al., 1998). Some may be construed as early misdiagnoses, but the veracity of the others as symptomatic ALS can be tested only with further research. An example is the concept of paraneoplastic ALS in carcinoma (Evans et al., 1990) and whether the association is coincidental or causal (Forsyth et al., 1997).

On the other hand, historical descriptions of lead intoxication, other heavy metal intoxications, Lyme disease, and hyperparathyroidism mimicking ALS have prompted innumerable tests searching for these diseases in the work-up of patients with ALS. Yet, after years of searching, it is now the consensus in large centers that these disorders virtually never simulate ALS. These may be construed as chance associations with ALS.

Other rare disorders may include amyotrophy in the context of hexosaminidase deficiency, multisystem atrophy, Parkinsonism dementia, and spinocerebellar ataxias, but the later development of distinguishing signs and symptoms makes it clear that the diagnosis is not classical ALS. In hexosaminidase deficiency especially, the superimposition of ataxia, corticospinal tract disorder, movement disorders, dementia, or psychiatric symptoms on top of lower motor neuron disease may understandably obscure the overall diagnosis. These may be construed as ALS as a symptom within a complex neurodegenerative disease, sometimes called 'MND-plus syndromes'.

By contrast, it is well reported that motor neuron disease is over-represented in patients with lymphoproliferative disorders (Schold et al., 1979; Openshaw and Slatkin, 1998; and see especially the work of the Columbia University group, Gordon et al., 1997). In Hodgkin's disease alone, the prevalence of MND has been estimated as 1%, which is 1000 times the prevalence of MND in the general population (Openshaw and Slatkin, 1998). In lymphoproliferative disorders, the MND is most often exclusively lower motor neuron in nature (Schold et al., 1979; Openshaw and Slatkin, 1998), but may be confused by soft upper motor neuron signs or even associated with definite upper motor neuron signs (Gordon et al., 1997). It often has a more subacute course than typical sporadic ALS. The temporal course of the MND seems not to follow the course of the underlying neoplasm (Schold et al., 1979), as it may be the presentation of lymphoma or occur very late in remission. Some series emphasize the benignity of the MND (Schold et al., 1979) whereas others emphasize the lethality of the MND and the rare response to therapy of the underlying malignancy (Gordon et al., 1997). The CSF protein is often over 70 mg/dl. This rather strong disease association implies either an immunologic disorder in a small subset of ALS or some, as yet unknown, shared cellular feature of lymphocytes and motor neurons.

The false positive diagnosis of ALS

Mulder (1980) was one of the first to call attention to the problem of how frequently other diseases are mistaken as ALS. Beginning with the observation that there is no single 'laboratory marker that will identify or even confirm the diagnosis', he found it 'not surprising that mistakes in diagnosis are made' and that 'even the most competent clinician may overlook the diagnosis or, more seriously, make an incorrect diagnosis.' Mulder reported a series of 46 consecutive patients in whom the diagnosis of ALS was mistakenly made at another center (see Table 2.1). The 46 included the following surprising array of diagnoses: cervical spondylosis, monomelic amyotrophy of upper extremities, inflammatory neuropathy, benign fasciculations with minimal atrophy, myopathy, multiple sclerosis, Shy–Drager syndrome, parkinsonism, arsenical myelopathy, lumbar spinal stenosis, multiple lacunar infarcts of the brain, brain tumor, brachial plexus neuropathy, foramen magnum tumor, syringomyelia, basilar invagination, and cervical cord meningioma. It is noteworthy that of the four patients with presumptive ALS who had only fasciculations three were physicians, mirroring the high frequency of benign fasciculations in paramedical personnel (Reed and Kurland, 1963).

Some commentators may trivialize such personal case collections as reflecting merely the inexperience of referring physicians or the biases of the authors. The problem in understanding the significance of such series, of course, is that one does not know the denominator of patients from whom these were selected for referral, and that one cannot assess fully the ascertainment bias based on the specific type of referral practice. Nevertheless, Mulder's series from the Mayo Clinic no doubt came from many hundreds of referred patients. The point is not the frequency of mistaken diagnoses but rather what we can learn from the diagnoses that can mimic ALS in the eyes of even seasoned clinicians.

Table 2.1 Misdiagnoses in ALS

Authors	Type of series	Number of patients referred as ALS	Number of erroneous diagnoses	%	Common misdiagnoses*
Belsh and Schiffman (1990; 1996)	Records review	33	14	43	False-negative diagnoses of ALS (commonly cervical stenosis)
	E-mail questionnaire	64	17	27	False-negative diagnoses of ALS
Mulder, 1980	Referral	—	46	—	False-positive diagnoses of ALS instead of cervical stenosis (12), monomelic amyotrophy (9), inflammatory neuropathy (5), benign fasciculations (4), myopathy (3), multiple sclerosis (2), foramen magnum tumor, syringomyelia, basilar invagination, cervical cord meningioma shy–Drager syndrome, parkinsonism, arsenic myelopathy, lumbar stenosis, multiple lacunar infarcts, brain tumor, brachial plexopathy
Kuncl (this series)	Referral	160	24	14	False-positive diagnoses of ALS instead of: cervical and lumbar spondylotic amyotrophy (9; one with spondylolisthesis; one with familial metaphyseal dysplasia), paraprotein-associated motor neuropathy (3), brachial plexopathy (2), monomelic amyotrophy, caffeine toxicity, multifocal motor neuropathy, spinobulbar muscular atrophy, jugular foramen schwannoma, myelopathy, adult-onset spinal muscular atrophy, polyneuropathy, myasthenia gravis, polymyositis
Traynor et al. 2000	Registry	437	32	7.3	False-positive diagnoses of ALS instead of: multifocal motor neuropathy (7), spinobulbar muscular atrophy (4), motor neuropathy (3), noncompressive myelopathy (2), spinal muscular atrophy (2), cervical spondylotic myelopathy, hereditary spastic paraparesis, postpolio syndrome, multiple sclerosis, hyperthyroidism, Pancoast syndrome, uncertain (8)
Davenport et al., 1996	Registry	552	46	8.3	False-positive diagnoses of ALS instead of: cervical spondylotic myeloradiculopathy (10), multiple strokes (5), multisystem atrophy (4), multiple sclerosis (4), radiculopathies (4), peripheral neuropathy (4), multifocal motor neuropathy (2), normal

				pressure hydrocephalus, retropharyngeal tumor, cervical meningioma, cranial mononeuropathy, benign fasciculations, brachial neuritis, ulnar neuropathy, lumbar stenosis, polymyositis, uncertain (4)	
Parboosingh et al., 1997	Referral[†]	147 (SALS) 100 (FALS) 20 (suspected SBMA)	3 5 7	2 5 35	ALS diagnosed instead of spinobulbar muscular atrophy

* Number in parentheses refers to number of patients; otherwise one patient per diagnosis
[†]All patients were male and had initially carried the diagnosis of definite to suspected ALS by the criteria of Swash and Leigh (1992) at major ALS centers. The 20 suspected of having spinobulbar muscular atrophy were originally diagnosed with ALS

Mulder's experience was mirrored in our own series of prospectively studied patients who were referred for electromyography or participation in clinical trials with a suspected diagnosis of ALS (see Table 2.1). Of 160 patients referred with that diagnosis, 24 turned out eventually not to have ALS. Spondylotic amyotrophy again topped the list, and electromyographic assessment of the thoracic paraspinal muscles turned out to be most helpful in the differential diagnosis early on in the disease (Kuncl et al., 1988). Some misdiagnoses, such as peripheral neuropathy, myasthenia gravis, and polymyositis, no doubt represent the subjective misinterpretation of previous electrodiagnostic data. Others may represent the chance superimposition of unrelated clinically 'silent' upper motor neuron signs upon a new, progressive lower motor neuron disorder of the motor unit which is not ALS. Still others are surprising. Nevertheless, these illustrative cases can especially teach us about the appropriate, sparing use of imaging and lumbar puncture in early diagnosis. Three are presented here.

Illustrative cases

Case 1

A 60-year-old man was referred to confirm the diagnosis of ALS. Two years earlier, painless weakness had begun in his right shoulder and had progressed gradually while the proximal shoulder muscles had atrophied. Eventually, at the point when he could just oppose gravity with his right arm, he developed some neck pain which did not radiate. Extension worsened the pain but it was controlled with aspirin. He had no numbness or symptoms referable to bowel or bladder. EMG had revealed acute and chronic partial denervation in the right arm and both legs but no sensory conduction abnormality, and the diagnosis of probable ALS had been made.

Twenty years previously he had lumbar spine surgery because of radiating back and leg pain and leg cramps, and recently his leg cramps had increased. He carried the diagnosis of 'osteoarthritis' because of finger deformities.

On examination, the right scapula was winged and he had wasting and weakness of rhomboids and serratus anterior on that side. The right biceps, deltoid, supraspinatus, wrist extensors – all having C5 or C6 input – were quite weak and wasted. A similar pattern of weakness was present on the left side but was less severe. The infraspinatus, triceps, and wrist flexors were normal. The right abductor pollicis brevis was slightly weak, but other intrinsic hand muscles were normal. In the legs, there was a symmetrical, upper motor neuron pattern of mild weakness in the bilateral iliopsoas and extensor hallucis but asymmetrical weakness and wasting of the extensor digitorum brevis muscles. The deep tendon reflexes were preserved, except for the right biceps. He had bilateral Hoffman signs, increased tone in the legs, but no Babinski signs and no jaw jerk. Pin and light touch sensation were normal, but he had threshold changes to vibratory sensation in the toes, ankles, fingers and wrists. The cranial nerves were normal.

He had multiple skeletal deformities. The spine appeared rigid and he held his neck stiffly. He had pectus carinatum. The bones of the shoulders, frontal bones of the skull, wrists, elbows, and all the joints of the hands and toes appeared quite enlarged. Cervical kyphosis and thoracolumbar scoliosis were moderate. It was discovered that three of his five siblings, all three of his children, his mother, and several maternal cousins had similarly deformed hands.

Sensory and motor conduction studies were normal. Needle EMG of arm muscles revealed the combination of fibrillation potentials, fasciculations, complex repetitive discharges and reduced recruitment in limb and paraspinal muscles limited to C5/6 roots bilaterally, matching the examination. EMG of the leg muscles was normal, except for minor denervation changes in the wasted extensor digitorum brevis muscles.

CT scan of the cervical spine showed moderately severe degenerative disk disease from C2 through C6, with disk narrowing and osteophyte formation, 4 mm of anterior subluxation of C2 on C3, kyphosis of the upper cervical spine, and narrowing of the upper cervical spinal canal in its anterior/posterior dimension (Figure 2.1). Similar degenerative changes were seen in the lumbar spine. More importantly, multiple bone radiographs evidenced multiple metaphyseal dysplasia (Pyle's familial dysplasia) as follows: thickened pubic rami and ischium, under-tubulation of the metaphyseal regions of the proximal femurs and humeri, short metacarpals and metatarsals with broad metaphyseal regions, and decreased thoracic and lumbar vertebral body height.

Follow-up exam 4 years later revealed that his right arm strength had improved after cervical spine decompression.

Diagnosis Combined cervical and lumbar spondylotic amyotrophy in familial metaphyseal dysplasia.

(a)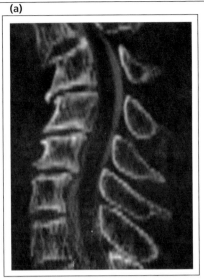

(b)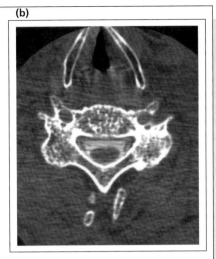

Fig. 2.1 Cervical stenosis in familial dysplasia simulating ALS (*Case 1*). CT scan of the cervical spine shows narrowing of the upper cervical spinal canal in its anterior/posterior dimension. This extended from C2 to C6 and was accompanied also by degenerative changes. (a) Lateral view; (b) transverse view at C5,6

Teaching principles To be definitive, upper motor neuron signs must occur in or rostral to weak wasted muscles, not merely in the same limb. Slowly progressing cervical spine compression over multiple high segments, especially if maximal in the anterior/posterior dimension, may produce both upper and lower motor neuron signs in the same limb in the absence of sensory changes, and may therefore simulate ALS when combined with a similar process in the lumbar spine. The frequency of spondylotic amyotrophy in the same age group as in ALS makes this a common differential diagnosis.

Case 2

Because of progressive left shoulder and tongue weakness a 53-year-old man presented for a second opinion on the diagnosis of ALS. A year and a half before he had noticed trouble whistling and then realized while brushing his teeth that the left side of his tongue was smaller than the right. Speech became slightly slurred. Some time later, during aerobic exercises, he developed occasional aching in the left shoulder 'of the type one gets when exercising to excess a weak muscle.' He noted that the muscle bulk around the left shoulder was reduced. In recent months, the shoulder weakness progressed. He then noticed that his voice became a little weaker and somewhat breathy in quality. Swallowing became somewhat difficult for solids and liquids and was accompanied by occasional coughing after eating or drinking, suggesting aspiration. He reported no fasciculation, muscle cramping, numbness, stiffness, bowel or bladder symptoms, nor motor dysfunction outside the upper left arm.

At the time of first presentation, one year into the course of his disease, an MRI of the brain showed only empty sella and a solitary punctate white matter intensity in the centrum semiovale.

Past history included narcolepsy, intermittent lumbosacral radicular pain, and breast reduction surgery on the right side. Family history was not revealing of neuromuscular disease.

General physical examination was unrevealing. Neurological exam was striking for severe furrowing and wasting of the left side of the tongue, which deviated to the left but did not fasciculate (Figure 2.2(a)). The remainder of the cranial nerve exam was normal. The muscles of the left shoulder, including trapezius, supraspinatus, and infraspinatus (all of which were mildly weak), appeared small but had no fasciculations. The left pectoral region appeared smaller than the right. By quantitative dynamometric testing comparing with the right side, the left deltoid was 40% decreased and the left biceps and triceps were 20% decreased. Remaining musculature of the other three limbs was normal. The jaw jerk was normal, but the tendon reflexes were brisk at biceps, triceps, and brachioradialis, more brisk on the left than the right. There were bilateral crossed adductor responses and a left extensor plantar response. Sensation, coordination, and gait were normal.

EMG showed fibrillations and positive sharp waves in the left tongue, but there were none elsewhere in the proximal or distal arm and leg muscles.

A second MRI scan with gadolinium contrast and with attention to the base of the skull revealed a 2-cm, rounded, well demarcated mass involving the lower part of the left jugular foramen and poststyloid parapharyngeal space (Figure 2.2(b,c)). At surgery, the mass was a circumscribed tumor situated medial to the left internal jugular vein and posterior to the internal carotid artery. The mass was contiguous with the vagus nerve. The hypoglossal nerve could not be separated from the tumor. Resection of the tumor was complete, but both the affected cranial nerves had to be divided. The histopathological diagnosis was schwannoma. Six years later, the patient's tumor had slowly recurred at the jugular foramen, and he had required a thyroplasty to correct dysphonia and aspiration.

Diagnosis Jugular foramen syndrome; schwannoma.

Teaching principles The diagnosis of ALS is semiologic and is therefore one of exclusion. Tongue dysfunction is most often upper motor neuron and bilateral in ALS; at the time of first diagnosis in ALS the cranial muscles are denervated in only a quarter of patients (Kuncl et al., 1988).

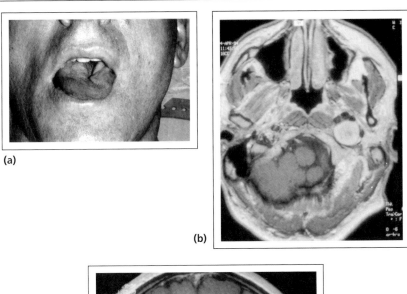

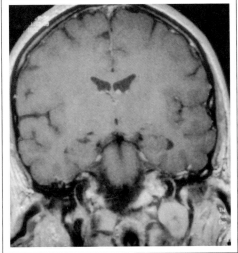

Fig. 2.2 Jugular foramen schwannoma simulating ALS (*Case 2*). (a) Furrowed, wasted left side of tongue; (b, c) A 2-cm mass involves the lower part of the left jugular foramen and poststyloid parapharyngeal space, medial to the internal jugular vein and posterior to the internal carotid artery. The mass is contiguous with the Xth and XIIth cranial nerves

Severe asymmetrical tongue atrophy suggests a focal lesion. Upper motor neuron signs must be rostral to the lower motor neuron signs, according to established diagnostic criteria (WFN Research Group on Neuro-muscular Diseases, 1998); upper motor neuron signs may also represent a 'silent' second disorder, in this case presumably cervical spondylosis. Two years of progression with no sign above the foramen magnum requires that a focal lesion be ruled out by imaging.

Case 3

A 61-year-old man with a history of progressive difficulty walking up stairs was referred with the diagnosis of probable ALS. As he considered himself a sportsman, having played American football, basketball, and baseball competitively in college and semi-professional baseball after college, he thought it was unusual that for the past 1 1/2 years he could not carry heavy objects up stairs and needed to use a bannister all the time. This progressed; he could not arise from a squat and began walking more slowly even on flat surfaces. An EMG had shown widespread denervation, and an MRI scan of the neck had been normal; hence the concern was that this was ALS.

He had minimized symptoms of progressive arm weakness by attributing it to age or a decades-old shoulder separation. Over the past several years, he was weaker pounding a nail and had difficulty lifting two cement blocks or a suitcase. Whereas 4 years earlier he had been able to do 30 push-ups, he could not do any in the past month.

Recently, dry food was swallowed more slowly, and he took longer to eat. Pronunciation and phonation were not changed. His wife noticed that when he was relaxed and not paying attention to it, his jaw slacked open. In retrospect, there had been a great deal of difficulty with his face. He was aware of bilateral twitching in the facial muscles for many years, perhaps as many as 10. For 4 years his eyes teared more (he was unaware of failure of tight eye closure). At a New Year's celebration a year ago, he recognized that he could no longer blow up a balloon or blow out an elongating noise maker although he had no trouble breathing.

The family history was pertinent only for a wheelchair-bound maternal first cousin (male) who died at 65 of a progressive ataxic disorder with onset in his 20s, which was thought to be spinocerebellar ataxia.

The general physical examination was unrevealing. He had no gynecomastia, but had creases above his pectoralis muscles, indicating long-term wasting.

He was unaware of his abnormal facial expression, which indicated longstanding weakness. His smile was transverse, and he could barely approximate the eyelids. He could approximate the lips, but without much pressure. The platysma contracted weakly. The tongue did not fasciculate at rest, had normal bulk, and was strong. Speech was normal. Muscle bulk was reduced bilaterally in the quadriceps, pectoralis, and biceps. Manual motor testing showed MRC 4–4+ strength in all muscles of the arms and proximal muscles of the legs. Fasciculations were seen in all four limbs, the rectus abdominus, and facial muscles. Deep tendon reflexes were present but required reinforcement. The jaw jerk was normal. The tone in the legs seemed increased, but there were no upper motor neuron signs. Pin and vibration sensation in the toes and hands were normal.

Examination of family photos revealed that facial weakness went back at least two decades.

Although the sural nerve potentials were reportedly normal 6 months previously when the diagnosis of ALS was made, the EMG/NCS now showed absent sural nerve potentials and reduced amplitude sensory potentials in the median, ulnar, and radial nerves (Figure 2.3). Amplitudes of the compound motor action potentials were at the lower limit of normal everywhere, but motor conduction velocities were normal. Virtually every limb and facial muscle examined by needle EMG had chronic partial denervation and decreased recruitment. Positive sharp waves were seen in the gastrocnemius and rectus abdominis. The serum CK was elevated twofold over the upper limit of normal. DNA testing revealed 41 CAG repeats in the Kennedy allele (normal, 11–33).

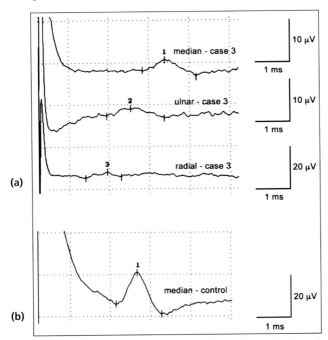

Fig. 2.3 Spinobulbar muscular atrophy (Kennedy disease) simulating ALS (*Case 3*). Across the board reduction in amplitudes of sensory nerve action potentials in this patient (a) compared with a control with radiculopathy (b) indicates that the disorder is a neuronopathy

Diagnosis Spinobolbar muscular atrophy (Kennedy syndrome).

Teaching principles Weakness with the patient unaware implies a very long history. Onset in males in the 30s or 40s is common in Kennedy syndrome but occurs in less than 20% of patients with ALS. Even though ALS may frequently begin with exclusively lower motor neuron signs, that presentation, or lower motor neuron disease with soft upper motor neuron signs, requires special attention to the differential diagnosis of disorders which are treatable or have quite different prognoses (Figure 2.4).

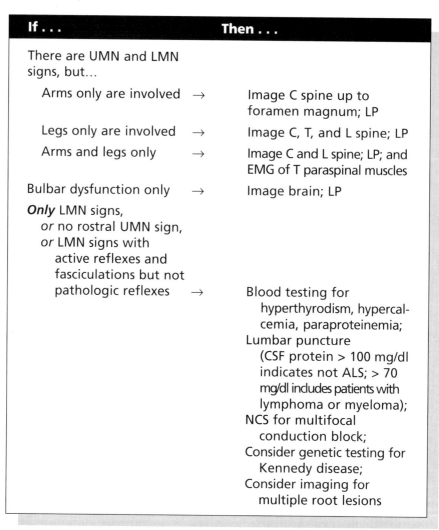

If . . .		Then . . .
There are UMN and LMN signs, but...		
Arms only are involved	→	Image C spine up to foramen magnum; LP
Legs only are involved	→	Image C, T, and L spine; LP
Arms and legs only	→	Image C and L spine; LP; and EMG of T paraspinal muscles
Bulbar dysfunction only	→	Image brain; LP
Only LMN signs, or no rostral UMN sign, or LMN signs with active reflexes and fasciculations but not pathologic reflexes	→	Blood testing for hyperthyrodism, hypercal-cemia, paraproteinemia; Lumbar puncture (CSF protein > 100 mg/dl indicates not ALS; > 70 mg/dl includes patients with lymphoma or myeloma); NCS for multifocal conduction block; Consider genetic testing for Kennedy disease; Consider imaging for multiple root lesions

Fig. 2.4 Practical use of imaging and lumbar puncture to reduce misdiagnosis in possible ALS. UMN, upper motor neuron; LMN, lower motor neuron; C, cervical; T, thoracic; L, lumbar; LP, lumbar puncture; NCS, nerve conduction studies

Patient registries

Patient registries – in which nearly full case ascertainment can be achieved in a relatively circumscribed region having a national health service, a well developed public health system, and a regional administration – may offer the clearest window on the true rate of misdiagnosis. This was attempted in the Republic of Ireland in the period 1993–1997 and by the Scottish MND Register from 1989 forward. In Ireland, a registry of 437 patients, representing virtually full ascertainment and a stable annual incidence of approximately 2.1/100,000 per year (Traynor et al., 1999), contained a false-positive diagnosis rate of 7.3% (Traynor et al., 2000). The most common mimicking conditions were multifocal motor neuropathy with conduction block and spinobulbar muscular atrophy. The experience in Scotland was much the same; the false-positive misdiagnosis rate was 8%, and half of those were potentially treatable (Davenport et al., 1996). The lowness of the figures in the Irish and Scottish registries compared with previous series, however, may reflect the fact that the appropriateness of diagnosis was judged rather late in the course of disease. In both registries the eventual diagnoses were clarified by the evolution of atypical symptoms excluding MND, the results of specific investigations, and the failure of symptoms to progress. The data of the Irish ALS Register illustrated that fully 84% of the misdiagnosed patients with an ALS mimic syndrome fulfilled the revised E1 Escorial criteria (WFN Research Group on Neuromuscular Diseases, 1994) for either 'suspected' or 'possible' ALS, 13% met the criteria for 'probable' ALS, and 3% for 'definite' ALS. The data from both registries allow the conclusion that the misdiagnosis of ALS still remains a common clinical problem despite modern investigations and greater sophistication about potential diagnostic pitfalls.

The special case of spinobulbar muscular atrophy

In the contemporary genetic era, DNA testing has amplified our understanding of the misdiagnosis of ALS. In a series derived from several centers (Parboosingh et al., 1997), 147 men who carried the diagnosis of sporadic ALS and 100 unrelated men with familial ALS were screened for CAG repeat expansions in the androgen receptor specific for spinobulbar muscular atrophy. The study revealed that the rate of misdiagnosis was 2%. Patients had been diagnosed as 'definite' or 'suspected' ALS according to the El Escorial criteria of 1992 (Swash and Leigh, 1992). It is clear that none of these patients could have or should have been given the appellation of *definite* ALS by the El Escorial criteria, as none of them had definite upper motor neuron signs. However, most of them lacked classic signs and symptoms of spinobulbar muscular atrophy, as most did not have gynecomastia, and minor sensory impairment was present in only half of the patients. The authors rightfully point out that the diagnosis of ALS is straightforward when a patient has all of the classic upper and lower motor neuron signs and symptoms of the disease yet they make the point well that the diagnosis of ALS is often entertained as 'suspected' or 'possible' before the development of all typical manifestations of the disease, often at the time when such a patient is seeking specialized treatment in an ALS center or referral to a clinical trial early in the course of the disease.

In ALS, more often than not, clinical and EMG signs reveal lower motor neuron dysfunction readily, but upper motor neuron signs are more equivocal. The absence of a family history, the absence of gynecomastia, or the absence of minimal sensory abnormalities are not sufficient to preclude a diagnosis of spinobulbar muscular atrophy. Minor intermittent sensory phenomena are often attributed to concurrent disease such as diabetes or entrapment neuropathy. Conversely, upper motor neuron signs in spinobulbar muscular atrophy may relate to a second neurologic disorder.

The distinction between the two diseases is obviously important because the prognosis for survival in spinobulbar muscular atrophy is normal, and the diagnosis also allows for genetic counseling of family members. The presence of a single unrecognized patient with spinobulbar muscular atrophy in a clinical trial which hopes to use survival as a primary outcome in ALS will be a problem, given the way that such trials are often constructed with marginal power.

Seasoned ALS experts who tend to see 'last resort' consultations late in disease can bet that these cases of unrecognized spinobulbar muscular atrophy would be atypical of ALS. However, that begs the question faced by the practicing clinician struggling with the differential diagnosis earlier in the course, when the patient's presentation may not be so typical, and when the pressure to begin therapy or enter a trial is great.

The false-negative diagnosis of ALS

Every seasoned clinician knows that, early on in its course, true ALS is often misdiagnosed as something else. In the USA, Belsh and Schiffman (1990; 1996) found that record reviews and e-mail surveys alike revealed a high rate of misdiagnosis (43% and 27%, respectively). This no doubt relates to the fact that patients were assessed very early rather than after disease progression, long duration of symptoms, and the elaboration of new signs, which can always make the 'last consultant the smartest' (Rowland, 1997). The fact that the rate of misdiagnosis was highest in urban patients and in those over the age of 60 can raise speculations about the biases of physicians regarding aging and the effect of abundant technology on the provision of medical care in cities. Again, as in the false-positive diagnosis of ALS, spinal stenosis/radiculopathy topped the list of causes.

Some would argue from a cost/benefit analysis that patients have little to gain from early diagnosis of ALS, given current treatment limitations (Smith, 2000). While this may seem true from a public policy perspective, few patients or doctors in the ALS community would agree. For most, delays in diagnosis do not merely delay inevitable existential awareness of fatal disease but delay practical action toward self education, planning one's future, gathering family emotional resources, participation in the currently available (though meager) neuroprotective therapies, and participation in meaningful therapeutic trial research.

Algorithm of indications for imaging and lumbar puncture

Given the above frequency and nature of erroneous diagnoses in ALS, one can derive an algorithm for the effective use of imaging and lumbar puncture in suspected ALS (Figure 2.4). This specific decision point amplifies the general diagnostic algorithm already presented in Chapter 1 (see Figure 1.1).

Erroneous diagnoses in spinal muscular atrophy

Unlike ALS, there is now a 'gold standard' for the diagnosis of most cases of SMA. The most common scenario is a diagnosis of what appears to be

Werdnig–Hoffman disease (acute, or type I SMA) that turns out with time to be a congenital myopathy. The most common mimics include severe X-linked nemaline myopathy, congenital fiber type disproportion, and other congenital myopathies. Occasionally, congenital myopathies are mistaken as childhood SMA (type II). One famous such mimic gained notoriety when a 28-year follow-up of what had been reported as the rare association of SMA with ophthalmoplegia turned out to be multiminicore myopathy (Gordon et al., 1996). For further discussion of the differential diagnosis of SMA, consult Chapter 5.

Significance and summary

It is obvious that false-positive diagnoses of ALS can have severe emotional consequences for the patient and may well destroy the patient–physician relationship. We have seen such cases go on to court proceedings in litiginous societies like the USA. The opposite problem, false-negative diagnoses of ALS, may at first seem less dismaying to some patients and physicians, but the consequences are nevertheless critical: delays in treatment, education, and entry into therapeutic trials.

The specific errant diagnoses masquerading as ALS can teach the clinician much about the pitfalls in diagnosis alluded to earlier in Chapter 1. They can become a list for differential diagnosis to improve the sophistication and helpfulness of the neurological consultation. Their frequency ranges from 7.3% to 43%, depending entirely on the referral nature of the practice and how early in the course of diagnosis the patient is seen. Closer case study of such patients can help mold an algorithm which can become a practical part of the clinician's approach to suspected motor neuron disease.

References

Belsh JM, Schiffman PL (1990) Misdiagnosis in patients with amyotrophic lateral sclerosis. Arch Intern Med 150: 2301–2305.

Belsh JM, Schiffman PL (1996) The amyotrophic lateral sclerosis (ALS) patient perspective on misdiagnosis and its repercussions. J Neurol Sci 139 (suppl) 100–116.

Davenport RJ, Swingler RJ, Chancellor AM, Warlow CP (1996) Avoiding false positive diagnoses of motor neuron disease: lessons from the Scottish Motor Neuron Disease Register. J Neurol Neurosurg Psychiatry 60: 147–151.

Evans BK, Fagan C, Arnold T, Dropcho EJ, Oh SJ (1990) Paraneoplastic motor neuron disease and renal cell carcinoma: improvement after nephrectomy. Neurology 40: 960–962.

Forsyth PA, Dalmau J, Graus F, Cwik V, Rosenblum MK, Posner JB (1997) Motor neuron syndromes in cancer patients. Ann Neurol 41: 722–730.

Gordon PH, Hays AP, Rowland LP et al. (1996) Erroneous diagnosis corrected after 28 years. Not spinal muscular atrophy with ophthalmoplegia but minicore myopathy. Arch Neurol 53: 1194–1196.

Gordon PH, Rowland LP, Younger DS et al. (1997) Lymphoproliferative disorders and motor neuron disease: an update. Neurology 48: 1671–1678.

Kuncl RW, Cornblath DR, Griffin JW (1988) Assessment of thoracic paraspinal muscles in the diagnosis of ALS. Muscle and Nerve 11: 484–492.

Mulder DW (1980) Commentary: Differential diagnosis of adult motor neuron diseases. In: Mulder DW (ed.) The Diagnosis and Treatment of Amyotrophic Lateral Sclerosis. Houghton Mifflin: Boston, pp. 79–82.

Openshaw H, Slatkin NE (1998) Motor neuron disease in Hodgkins lymphoma. Neurology 50: A31.

Parboosingh JS, Figlewicz DA, Krizus A et al. (1997) Spinobulbar muscular atrophy can mimic ALS: The importance of genetic testing in male patients with atypical ALS. Neurology 49: 568–572.

Reed DM, Kurland LT (1963) Muscle fasciculations in a healthy population. Arch Neurol 9: 363–367.

Ross MA, Miller RG, Berchert L et al. and the rhCNTF ALS Study Group (1998) Toward earlier diagnosis of amyotrophic lateral sclerosis: revised criteria. Neurology 50: 768–772.

Rowland, LP (1997) Diagnosis of amyotrophic lateral sclerosis. Abstracts, Eighth International Congress on ALS/MND, Glasgow, Scotland.

Salachas F, Lafitte C, Chassande B et al. (1998) Motor neuron disease mimicking amyotrophic lateral sclerosis or primary lateral sclerosis in primary Sjögren's syndrome. Neurology 50: A31.

Schold SC, Cho ES, Somasundaram M, Posner JB (1979) Subacute motor neuronopathy: a remote effect of lymphoma. Ann Neurol 3: 271–287.

Smith RA (2000) Effects of the early diagnosis of amyotrophic lateral sclerosis on the patient: disadvantages. ALS 1 (Suppl 1): S75–77).

Swash M, Leigh N (1992) Criteria for diagnosis of familial amyotrophic lateral sclerosis. Neuromuscular Disorders 2: 7–9.

Traynor BJ, Codd MB, Corr B, Forde C, Frost E, Hardiman O (1999) Incidence and prevalence of ALS in Ireland, 1995–1997: a population-based study. Neurology 52: 504–509.

Traynor BJ, Codd MB, Corr B, Forde C, Frost E, Hardiman O (2000) Amyotrophic lateral sclerosis mimic syndromes: a population-based study. Arch Neurol 57: 109–113.

World Federation of Neurology Research Group on Neuromuscular Diseases (1994) El Escorial World Federation of Neurology Criteria for the diagnosis of amyotrophic lateral sclerosis. J Neurol Sci 124 (Suppl): 96–107.

World Federation of Neurology Research Group on Motor Neuron Diseases (1998) El Escorial revisited: revised criteria for the diagnosis of amyotrophic lateral sclerosis. http://www.wfnals.org/Articles/elescorial1998.htm

3

Current concepts in the pathogenesis of ALS

Pamela J. Shaw and Ralph W. Kuncl

Amyotrophic lateral sclerosis (ALS) is one of the most common adult-onset human neurodegenerative disorders. The cell death process in ALS is relatively selective for lower motor neuron groups in the ventral horn of the spinal cord (Figure 3.1 (a, b)) and brainstem, and for upper motor neurons, a proportion of which are represented by the giant cells of Betz in the motor cortex. The selective vulnerability of motor neurons is relative, and there is now increasing evidence from clinical studies (Hattori, 1984; Subramanium and Yiannikas, 1990; Kew et al., 1993a,b; Chari et al., 1996) and pathological (Williams et al., 1995; Ince et al., 1996, 1998a,b; Iwanaga et al., 1997) that involvement outside the motor system commonly occurs in ALS (Figure 3.1 (c, d)). Thus ALS can be regarded as a multisystem disease in which the motor system is affected early and most severely. Even within motor neuron groups there is variation in the vulnerability to the neurodegenerative process. Certain groups of motor neurons tend to be relatively spared from injury in ALS, including those brainstem motor nuclei innervating extraocular muscles and those motor neurons in Onuf's nucleus of the sacral spinal cord which innervate the muscles of the pelvic floor. Comparison of cell specific neurochemical profiles in neuronal groups with differential vulnerability in ALS may provide important insights into the neurodegenerative process.

The primary pathogenetic processes underlying ALS are likely to be multifactorial, and the precise molecular pathways leading to cell death of motor neurons are at present unknown. Evidence is emerging to indicate that the neuronal injury in ALS reflects a complex interaction between genetic factors, imbalance of the glutamatergic neurotransmitter system, and oxidative stress, which may result in damage to critical target proteins and organelles (Coyle and Puttfarcken 1993; Olanow, 1993; Shaw, 1994; Zeman et al., 1994; Brown, 1995; Rothstein, 1995; Tu et al., 1996). In some patients with ALS immunological mechanisms may contribute to motor neuron injury (Appel et al., 1995; Smith and Appel 1995).

This chapter will review current concepts in the pathogenesis of ALS, with emphasis on recent neuroscientific developments. The potential contribution of genetic factors, dysfunction of the glutamatergic neurotransmitter system,

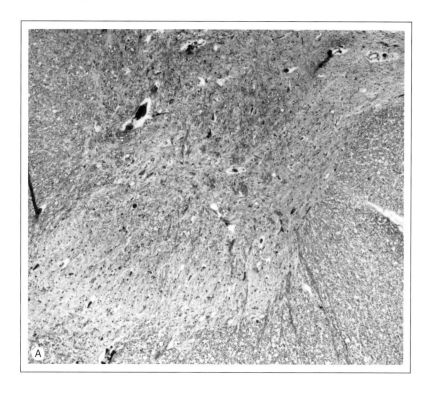

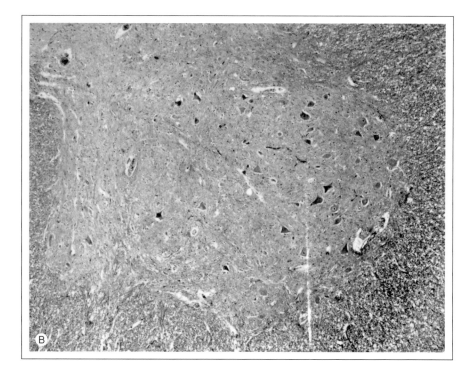

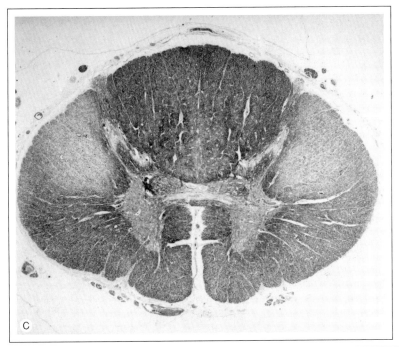

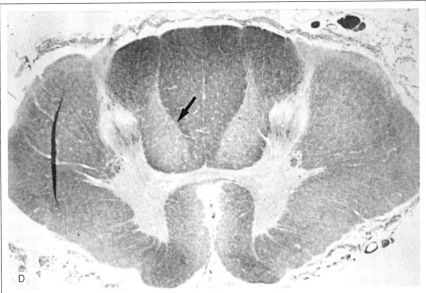

Fig. 3.1 The pathology of ALS. (A) Photomicrograph of lumbar spinal cord from a patient with ALS shows the mild shrinkage of gray matter and marked depletion of the large motor neurons in the anterior horn. (B) Compare with the normal density of anterior horn cells in a control subject. (A and B, hematoxylin–eosin.) (C) Spinal cord section from a patient with classical sporadic ALS, showing degeneration of the descending lateral corticospinal tracts and small anterior horns. Compare with (D), a patient carrying the E100G SOD1 mutation of familial ALS, showing pathological changes (abnormal myelin pallor; arrow) in the dorsal column sensory pathways as well as in the corticospinal pathways in the anterolateral white matter. (C and D, Luxol fast blue stain.) (A–C, adapted from Kuncl et al., 1992, with permission)

oxidative stress, and disturbance of intracellular calcium homeostasis in relation to motor neuron injury will be reviewed. Intracellular targets which may be most vulnerable in the process of motor neuron death, including mitochondria, neurofilament proteins, and several proteins which control glutamate neurotransmission, will also be discussed.

Genetic factors and ALS

The role of genetic factors in the etiology of ALS will be fully discussed in Chapter 4, and only a brief outline will be included here. ALS is sporadic in 90–95% and familial in approximately 5–10% of cases. Familial cases usually show autosomal dominant inheritance, though autosomal recessive inheritance may be seen, for example, in a Tunisian form of the disease. A major step forward in research into the underlying pathophysiology of ALS came from the discovery in 1993 that 20% of pedigrees with autosomal dominant familial ALS showed mutations in the gene on chromosome 21 that encodes the free radical scavenging enzyme Cu/Zn superoxide dismutase (SOD1) (Rosen et al., 1993). The genetic alterations underlying the remaining 80% of cases of autosomal dominant familial ALS remain to be uncovered. The autosomal recessive Tunisian form of ALS is linked to chromosome 2 (Hentati et al., 1994), but the responsible gene has not yet been identified. In rare cases of sporadic ALS, deletions or insertions in the gene encoding the neurofilament heavy subunit protein have been reported (Figlewicz et al., 1994; Tomkins et al., 1994). Isolated recent publications have reported mutations in the genes encoding the cytochrome c oxidase subunit 1, which is part of the terminal component of the mitochondrial respiratory chain (Comi et al., 1998), and the AP endonuclease enzyme, which is a key enzyme in the repair of oxidative damage to DNA (Olkowski, 1998). It has also been suggested that the apolipoprotein e4 genotype is a risk factor for the development of bulbar onset ALS (Al-Chalabi et al., 1996), though not all research groups have agreed on this finding.

Thus, genetic predisposition is clearly a very important factor in the etiology of ALS. Multiple different abnormal gene products can set the scene for motor neuron degeneration. Because of the clinical and pathological similarities between familial ALS and the more common sporadic form of the disease, insights gained from the investigation of the cellular consequences of genetic mutations may well improve our understanding of the process of cell death in sporadic ALS.

The glutamate neurotransmitter system in ALS

To facilitate critical appraisal of the evidence that dysfunction of the glutamate neurotransmitter system may contribute to motor neuron injury in ALS, it is appropriate to briefly review the normal process of glutamate neurotransmission, the current state of knowledge regarding the expression of glutamate receptor subtypes by human motor neurons, and the concept of excitotoxicity.

Normal glutamate neurotransmission

Glutamate is the major excitatory neurotransmitter in the human CNS (Figure 3.2). During normal glutamatergic neurotransmission glutamate is released from the presynaptic neuronal terminal and activates postsynaptic glutamate receptors. The excitatory signal is terminated by active removal of glutamate from the synaptic cleft by glutamate reuptake transporter proteins located predominantly on perisynaptic astrocytes. Aspartate, another excitatory amino

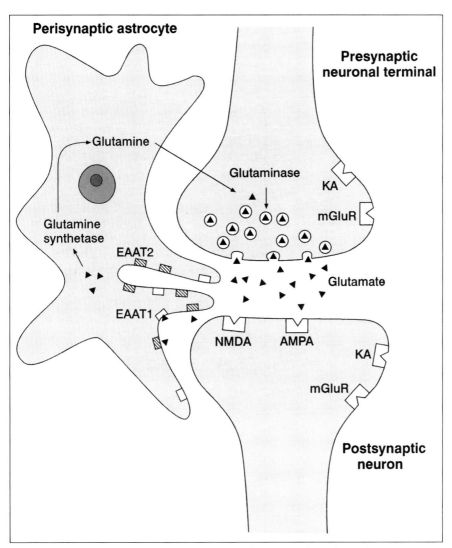

Fig. 3.2 Normal glutamatergic neurotransmission. Glutamate, released into the synaptic cleft, can activate several types of postsynaptic receptors (NMDA, AMPA, kainate, and metabotropic) before being actively removed by glutamate transporters (EAAT1 and EAAT2) located on perisynaptic astrocytes. Within glial cells, glutamate is converted to glutamine by the action of the enzyme glutamine synthetase. Glutamine is then shuttled back to the presynaptic neuron where it is converted back to glutamate by glutaminase. A modulatory role has been proposed for presynaptic metabotropic (mGluR) and kainate (KA) receptors

acid, is handled analogously and shares the same transporter. Neurotransmitter glutamate is recycled via the glutamate–glutamine cycle. Synaptic glutamate that has been transported into perisynaptic astrocytes is converted to glutamine by the enzyme glutamine synthetase. Glutamine is then transported back to the neuronal terminal where it is reconverted back to neurotransmitter glutamate by the action of glutaminase (Laake et al., 1995).

Postsynaptic glutamate receptors are divided into two major classes: ionotropic receptors which are ligand gated ion channels, and metabotropic receptors which are coupled through G proteins to intracellular second messenger systems (Westbrook, 1994). The ionotropic receptors are further subdivided into three major groups based on the pharmacological specificity of their selective agonists: N-methyl-D-aspartate (NMDA); α-amino-3-hydroxy-5-methyl-4-isoxazole propionic acid (AMPA); and kainate receptors. Fourteen different genes encoding ionotropic glutamate receptor subunits have now been identified (Hollman and Heinemann, 1994). In vivo, each functional receptor is thought to be formed from four or five subunits arranged as hetero-oligomers or possibly homo-oligomers. The physiologic properties of postsynaptic glutamate receptors depend on the specific combination of receptor subunits present in the receptor complex (Sommer and Seeburg, 1992). Further molecular and functional diversity arises from alternative splicing of the genes encoding receptor subunits and from posttranscriptional RNA editing (Hume et al., 1991; Burnashev et al., 1992). Clearly great potential diversity in the molecular structure of postsynaptic glutamate receptors can be generated from combinations of 14 gene products, and their splice variants, with or without additional RNA editing. There is therefore the potential for particular classes of neurons, such as motor neurons, to express a unique molecular profile of ionotropic glutamate receptors, suited to cell-specific functional properties.

Glutamatergic inputs to motor neurons arise from the descending corticospinal pathways (Young et al., 1983; Young and Penney, 1992), from collaterals of A-α fibers innervating muscle spindles and Golgi tendon organs (Molander et al., 1989; Burke, 1990), and from spinal cord excitatory interneurons (O'Brien and Fischbach, 1986).

In relation to the glutamate reuptake transport process, five human glutamate transporter genes have been cloned: excitatory amino acid transporter 1 (EAAT1) and EAAT2 are glial transporter proteins (Danbolt et al., 1992; Rothstein et al., 1994a; EAAT3 is localized to neurons (Rothstein et al., 1994b); EAAT4 is expressed mainly in the cerebellum (Fairman et al., 1995); and EAAT5 is localized to the retina (Arriza et al., 1997). Anti-sense knockdown and other studies suggest that EAAT2 is the functionally dominant transporter in terminating the excitatory glutamate mediated signal (Haugeto et al., 1996; Rothstein et al., 1996).

Glutamate receptor profile of human motor neurons

Human motor neurons have a high density of glutamate receptors (Shaw et al., 1991; Williams et al., 1996). Mammalian motor neurons in culture are susceptible to toxic effects following activation of either NMDA or nonNMDA receptors (Estevez et al., 1995). Autoradiographic studies with specific radioligands for NMDA, AMPA and kainate receptors in the human spinal cord, brainstem and motor cortex have confirmed that these receptor subtypes are present in the motor neuron areas (Shaw et al., 1991; Chinnery et al., 1993; Shaw and Ince, 1994). Labeling of NMDA receptors with [^{3}H-MK801] revealed focal areas of high intensity of binding in close proximity to the motor neuron perikarya (Shaw et al., 1991). Ligands for AMPA/kainate receptors show a more uniform labeling of the ventral horn gray matter (Chinnery et al., 1993; Shaw et al., 1994a,b). There are differences in the relative density of NMDA and nonNMDA receptor binding sites expressed by motor neuron groups which are vulnerable and nonvulnerable to the disease process in ALS (see below).

More recently, immunohistochemical studies using antibodies to specific glutamate receptor subunits have extended the findings obtained by autoradiography. Human motor neurons have a high level of expression of the universal NMDA receptor subunit, NMDAR1, and interestingly dendritic staining is much lighter than the staining of the cell body, which is unlike the pattern of staining seen in many other groups of neurons (Shaw, 1998). To date, there is little information on the expression of the eight splice variants of NMDAR1, and that of the NMDAR2A-2D subunits by human motor neurons. This information will be of interest because specific molecular features of NMDA receptor assembly may have important effects on cellular vulnerability to glutamate toxicity (Traynelis et al., 1995).

In relation to nonNMDA receptors, human spinal motor neurons and/or surrounding presynaptic processes show positive immunoreactivity with antibodies to the KA2 and GluR6/7 subunits (Shaw, 1998). Recent interesting data has emerged regarding the expression of AMPA receptor subunits by human motor neurons. AMPA receptors are composed of heteromeric complexes of four protein subunits, GluR1 to GluR4, and are responsible for much of the fast excitatory neurotransmission in the mammalian CNS. The GluR2 subunit has particular functional significance because, when incorporated into the AMPA receptor complex in its dominant edited form, the receptor is rendered impermeable to calcium (Burnashev et al., 1995). Most AMPA receptors in the human CNS include the edited GluR2 subunit and are therefore impermeable to calcium (Bettler and Mulle, 1995; Day et al., 1995). However, upper and lower motor neurons in the human CNS appear to have a very low or absent expression of GluR2 at both mRNA and protein level (Williams et al., 1997; Shaw et al., 1999). This means that AMPA receptors expressed by motor neurons are likely to be predominantly atypical and calcium permeable. The pathophysiological significance of the expression of calcium permeable AMPA receptors by particular cell groups has not yet been fully elucidated. However, calcium is known to play a crucial role in mediating toxic cellular events following glutamate receptor activation (Meldrum and Garthwaite, 1990). Neuronal subpopulations expressing AMPA receptors lacking the GluR2 subunit exhibit increased vulnerability to toxicity following activation by nonNMDA receptor agonists in vitro (Brorson et al., 1995). Thus, the molecular profile of AMPA receptors expressed by motor neurons could be one factor rendering this cell group vulnerable to glutamate-mediated toxicity.

Excitotoxicity

The excitatory action of glutamate, crucial for normal CNS function, can, if inadequately controlled, become transformed into a toxic action resulting in neuronal injury and death. The term *excitotoxicity* was coined to name this process (Olney, 1978). The details of the molecular mechanisms whereby glutamate damages neurons are still being elucidated, but several pathways which contribute to the toxic effects have been defined. Although most experimental work has focused on the role of glutamate in *acute* neuronal death, emerging lines of evidence indicate that cellular damage can accumulate over a longer time scale, the so-called 'slow' or 'weak' excitotoxicity (Susel et al., 1991; Rothstein et al., 1993).

Studies in vitro have shown two distict phases involved in excitotoxicity. First, depolarization-mediated influx of Na^+, Cl^- and water causes acute neuronal swelling which is reversible (Choi, 1987). Second, there is an influx of calcium, either directly through the ion channels of NMDA or calcium-permeable AMPA receptors or indirectly via activation of voltage-gated calcium channels (Miller et al., 1989). Under normal circumstances the intracellular calcium concentration is tightly controlled at a level below 0.1 µM. Regulation is maintained by a complex system of compartmentalization and transportation, involving sequestration within organelles such as the endoplasmic reticulum and mitochondria, binding to calcium binding proteins such as parvalbumin and calbindin D28K, and transport to the extracellular environment by ion exchangers (Baimbridge et al., 1992; Orrenius et al., 1989). The downstream consequences of excessive activation of cell surface glutamate receptors include destabilization of intracellular calcium homeostasis, with activation of a cascade of potentially injurious biochemical processes. Calcium-activated enzyme systems can damage the neuron both directly and through the generation of free radicals (Meldrum and Garthwaite, 1990).

Secondary excitotoxicity

The concept of secondary excitotoxicity may be particularly relevant as a contributory factor to neuronal death in chronic neurodegenerative diseases such as ALS. It is now apparent that excitotoxic cellular injury can occur as a secondary process triggered by a primary pathological event which results in compromised neuronal energy status (Novelli et al., 1988; Beal, 1993). Thus, impairment of neuronal glucose metabolism, mitochondrial dysfunction leading to reduced ATP production, or dysfunction of Na^+/K^+ ATPases will result in loss of the normal resting membrane potential of the cell. In this situation, there will be loss of the normal voltage-dependent Mg^{++} block of NMDA receptor channels, resulting in excessive activation of NMDA receptors by normal exposure to glutamate. A variety of primary disturbances in neuronal metabolism could predispose to secondary toxicity mediated by glutamate. When the process of secondary toxicity is operating, anti-glutamate therapy may be helpful in reducing neuronal injury, regardless of the primary pathophysiological process.

Oxidative glutamate toxicity

Oxidative glutamate toxicity is mediated via a series of disturbances to the redox homeostasis of the cell (Murphy et al., 1989; Maher and Davis, 1996). These pathways have not been completely characterized, but several processes may be important. Activation of glutamate receptors is an important pathway for the generation of intracellular free radicals via calcium-dependent activation of the arachidonic acid cascade, nitric oxide synthase and calpain (Lees, 1993; Pelligrini-Giampietro, 1994). Activation of both NMDA and nonNMDA receptor subtypes has been shown to directly stimulate the production of superoxide radicals (Bondy and Lee, 1993; Lafon-Cazal et al., 1993). Oxidative stress can cause damage to intracellular DNA, lipids and proteins, with the potential for cumulative dysfunction of essential organelles and macromolecules. Glutamate can also directly affect the ability of neurons to withstand oxidative stress by causing depletion of intracellular glutathione (Murphy et al., 1989).

Evidence for dysfunction of the glutamate neurotransmitter system in ALS

There is a body of circumstantial evidence implicating a disturbance of the glutamate neurotransmitter system as a contributory factor in the pathogenesis of motor neuron injury in ALS. This has been the subject of several recent reviews (Shaw et al., 1994; Zeman et al., 1994; Rothstein 1995; Leigh and Meldrum, 1996; Shaw and Ince, 1997).

Glutamate levels in CNS tissue, CSF, and plasma in ALS

Studies from several laboratories have shown a decrease in the level of glutamate in multiple regions of the CNS in postmortem tissue from ALS patients (Tsai et al., 1991). Perry et al. (1987) and Plaitakis et al. (1988) reported reduced levels of glutamate in both the brain and spinal cord of ALS patients. Malessa and coworkers identified decreased levels of glutamate in cervical and lumbar spinal cord, involving white as well as gray matter (Malessa et al., 1991).

In contrast, the levels of glutamate in CSF have been reported by several groups to be significantly elevated in ALS (Rothstein et al., 1990; Shaw et al., 1995a), though not all studies have confirmed this finding (Perry et al., 1990). There are technical difficulties in measuring glutamate levels in biological samples. This is exemplified by the finding that a 15-fold variation in the level of CSF glutamate has been reported in normal human controls from different laboratories. The levels of glutamate measured by automated HPLC are 10-fold lower than when measured by ion exchange chromatography (Rothstein et al., 1991). It also appears that the level of glutamate can vary with age and gender (Ferraro and Hare, 1985), so comparison groups need to be matched for these parameters. ALS patients may also be heterogeneous with respect to CSF glutamate. One recent study reported that the observed increase in CSF glutamate may be present in only 30% of ALS patients, the remainder having levels within the normal range (Shaw et al., 1995b). The CSF of ALS patients has been shown to be toxic to cultured neurons via activation of nonNMDA glutamate receptors (Couratier et al., 1993). However, it has not been demonstrated whether such toxicity correlates with the level of CSF glutamate.

Conflicting results have been reported in relation to fasting plasma glutamate levels in ALS patients. Plaitakis and Caroscio (1987) reported that fasting plasma glutamate levels are approximately doubled in ALS patients, and that oral glutamate loading produces abnormally high plasma levels in ALS patients compared with controls. Other groups, however, have failed to replicate these findings and have reported a normal profile of plasma amino acids in ALS patients (Rothstein et al., 1990; Shaw et al., 1995a). Therefore, the available data on CSF and plasma glutamate in ALS are conflicting and could not, by themselves, provide unequivocal evidence for or against the glutamatergic hypothesis of motor neuron injury.

Glutamate reuptake transporters in ALS

There is evidence that the expression and function of the glial glutamate transporter system, responsible for removing glutamate from the synaptic cleft and terminating the excitatory signal, may be abnormal in ALS. Such a defect could potentially give rise to an elevation in the level of extracellular glutamate and thus to excitotoxic neuronal injury. The first indication was a specific defect in the synaptosomal Na^+-dependent glutamate uptake in postmortem spinal cord and pathologically affected areas of brain from ALS patients (Rothstein et al., 1992). An autoradiographic study subsequently showed a reduction in $[^3H]$-D-aspartate binding to the glutamate reuptake transporter system in ALS spinal cord (Shaw et al., 1994c). Subsequent studies investigated the expression of glutamate transporter proteins in the CNS, with results which have not been entirely concordant. Immunoblotting studies performed on CNS tissue homogenates using anti-peptide polyclonal antibodies to glutamate transporter proteins showed a substantially reduced expression of the glial transporter protein EAAT2 in the motor cortex and spinal cord of ALS cases (Rothstein et al., 1995). The mean level of EAAT2 immunoreactivity in the motor cortex was decreased by 70%, and in approximately 25% of cases the expression of the protein was almost completely lost, whereas the expression of another glial protein, glial fibrillary acidic protein, was preserved. Fray et al. (1998) subsequently examined the expression of the EAAT2 protein in situ using immunohistochemistry and a monoclonal antibody produced to human recombinant EAAT2 protein. This study showed no reduction in the expression of EAAT2 in the motor cortex; indeed a slight increase was observed in the middle laminae. However, a significant decrease in EAAT2 immunoreactivity was observed in all gray matter regions of the lumbar spinal cord in ALS patients compared with controls. The differences between these two studies may be due to differences in the antigenic specificity of the antibodies employed, differences in tissue retrieval and storage, and the potential instability of EAAT2 in tissue extracts. However, both studies provide evidence for an alteration in EAAT2 expression in ALS, and further investigation is required to establish the underlying mechanism. It is of interest that the EAAT2 protein is known to be particularly vulnerable to damage by oxidative stress (Volterra et al., 1992). It is also of interest that reduced expression of the GLT-1 protein (equivalent to human EAAT2) (Bruijn et al., 1997) and decreased function of the high-affinity Na^+-dependent transport of glutamate in synaptosomal preparations (Canton et al., 1998) have been reported in transgenic mice with ALS-related

SOD1 mutations. This suggests that alteration in glutamate transporter expression may occur secondarily to other primary pathophysiological processes.

There is no evidence that genomic mutations in *EAAT2 commonly* underlie familial or sporadic ALS (Aoki et al., 1998). However, a spontaneous mutation of EAAT2 in a single patient with sporadic ALS provides the proof of principle that a genetically altered glutamate transporter can likely contribute to the excitotoxicity that participates in motor neuron degeneration (Trotti et al., 2001). The mutation, a substitution of an asparagine by a serine residue at the putative N-glycosylation site (N206S), was shown in oocyte expression studies to reduce glycosylation of EAAT2 and its insertion into plasmalemma, to decrease glutamate uptake, and to worsen the propensity of the transporter to reverse its direction of function under adverse conditions. As the mutation was heterozygous, it was important to demonstrate by co-expression studies that it exerted a dominant negative effect on wild type transporter EAAT2 (Trotti et al., 2001).

At the mRNA level there appears to be no alteration in the overall amount of *EAAT2* expression (or message) in ALS, as demonstrated by northern blotting (Bristol and Rothstein, 1996). Initially, one report described multiple abnormal mRNA transcripts, including exon-skipping and intron-retention splice variants (Lin et al., 1998). These abnormal transcripts were allegedly found in 65% of ALS cases, but not in controls, and were apparently confined to pathologically affected areas of CNS tissue, as well as being detectable in the CSF. In vitro expression studies suggested that proteins translated from these abnormal *EAAT2* transcripts have increased susceptibility to degradation and may exert a dominant negative effect on the expression and function of the normal EAAT2 protein. It was suggested that these variant mRNAs might result from gene-specific RNA processing errors, confined to particular anatomical sites in the CNS, and that this novel mechanism might be of fundamental importance in the pathogenesis of ALS. As yet, there is no clear explanation as to why such aberrant RNA processing might only affect *EAAT2* pre-mRNA and why only in the motor cortex and spinal cord. However, subsequent reports have suggested that alternatively spliced forms of *EAAT2* mRNA are not at all specific to ALS and can also be detected in both normals and neurodegenerative disease controls, including Alzheimer's disease and Lewy body disease (Nagai et al., 1998; Honig et al., 1999; Flowers et al., 2001). Therefore, it appears that aberrant processing of mRNA for the EAAT2 protein does not play a role in the pathophysiology of ALS and that the original report was in error, as it did not include sufficient neurodegenerative disease controls. An alternative explantion for disturbed glutamate homeostasis in ALS must be sought.

Whether a primary or secondary mechanism, reduced efficiency of glutamate clearance from the vicinity of motor neurons could still contribute to the cascade of motor neuron injury. It is of interest that lower motor neuron groups vulnerable in ALS, such as spinal motor neurons, have a much higher perisomatic expression of the EAAT2 protein than motor neuron groups such as the oculomotor neurons, which are less vulnerable to the disease process (Milton et al., 1997) (Figure 3.3).

Alteration of glutamate receptor expression and function in ALS

Autoradiographic studies have shown an increased density of binding sites for NMDA and non-NMDA receptor ligands in ALS, particularly in the

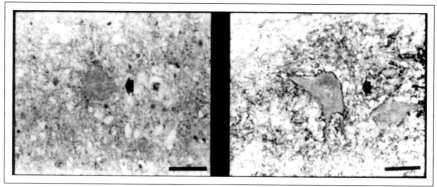

Fig. 3.3 The expression of the glutamate transporter protein EAAT2 in relation to motor neurons in the normal CNS. There is a much greater perisomatic expression of EAAT2 in the vicinity of spinal motor neurons (right), which are vulnerable to the disease process in ALS, compared to oculomotor neurons (left), which tend to be spared in ALS

intermediate gray matter of the spinal cord and in the deep layers of the motor cortex (Shaw et al., 1994a,b). It is possible that this represents an increased excitatory drive to surviving motor neurons in a failing motor system, but it may also contribute to the cascade of neuronal injury in ALS.

Abnormal excitability of the motor system in ALS patients has also been demonstrated in life. Positron emission tomography (PET) scanning studies have shown abnormally widespread activation of several contralateral cortical regions, following freely selected upper limb movements (Kew et al., 1993b). This implies an inappropriate activation of neurons outside the somatotopic representation of the upper limb, suggesting an imbalance between cortical excitatory and inhibitory neurotransmission in individuals with ALS. Transcranial magnetic stimulation of the motor cortex in ALS has shown abnormalities in a proportion of patients reflecting the presence of hyperexcitability of motor neurons (Eisen et al., 1993; Mills, 1995).

Anti-glutamate therapy in ALS and in animal models of the disease

The anti-glutamate agent riluzole modestly improves survival, both in ALS patients (Bensimon et al., 1994; Lacomblez et al., 1996) and in mutant SOD1 transgenic mice (Gurney et al., 1996). Riluzole interferes with pre- and post-synaptic glutamate neurotransmission via a complex mechanism of action involving blockade of voltage-sensitive Na^+ channels, ionic flux through NMDA channels and possibly also by interaction with G proteins (Doble et al., 1992; Debono et al., 1993; Hubert et al., 1994). Riluzole inhibits glutamate release, decreases excitatory amino acid evoked firing of rat facial motor neurons, and exerts neuroprotective effects in experimental models of acute and chronic neurodegenerative diseases (Girdlestone et al., 1989; Malgouris et al., 1994; Estevez et al., 1995; Rothstein and Kuncl, 1995). A potentially important property of riluzole is that it has dramatically higher affinity for the inactivated compared to the activated state of Na^+ channels (Hebert et al., 1994). This state-dependent drug affinity means that riluzole can be expected to preferentially block depolarized, hyperactive neurons.

Susceptibility of motor neurons to glutamate toxicity

To be plausible, the 'glutamate hypothesis' of motor neuron injury must explain how motor neurons could be selectively damaged by a disturbance of the glutamate neurotransmitter system, given that glutamate receptors have a widespread distribution throughout the CNS.

Mammalian motor neurons in culture have been shown to be susceptible to toxic effects following activation of either NMDA or nonNMDA glutamate receptors (Estevez et al., 1995). Intrathecal injection of the excitatory amino acid agonist kainic acid preferentially injures anterior horn cells in mice and induces the formation of abnormally phosphorylated neurofilaments, a cytoskeletal abnormality that has been documented in ALS (Hugon and Vallat, 1990). Organotypic rat spinal cord explants maintained in culture under conditions of pharmacological blockade of glutamate reuptake exhibit neurotoxicity which appears relatively selective for motor neurons (Rothstein et al., 1993).

Two cell-specific molecular features of human motor neurons have been identified which may render this cell group unduly susceptible to calcium-mediated toxic events following glutamate receptor activation. The first feature is the low/absent expression of the GluR2 AMPA receptor subunit and the resulting probability that human motor neurons express predominantly atypical, calcium-permeable AMPA receptors, as discussed earlier in this chapter (Williams et al., 1997). The second feature is that human motor neurons vulnerable to neurodegeneration in ALS lack the intracellular expression of the calcium-binding proteins parvalbumin and calbindin D28k (Ince et al., 1993). These proteins buffer intracellular calcium and may play an important role in the protection of neurons from calcium-mediated injury following glutamate receptor activation. A direct relationship has been shown between neuronal calcium buffering capacity and resistance to glutamate neurotoxicity (Mattson et al., 1989). These two molecular features may render human motor neurons differentially susceptible to calcium toxicity following AMPA receptor activation and begin to provide a plausible explanation of how disturbance of glutamatergic neurotransmission may cause selective injury to motor neurons.

Oxidative stress in ALS

Mechanism

Free radicals are a potential source of damage to proteins, DNA, lipids and membranes within cells. A state of oxidative stress exists when there is an imbalance between intracellular production of free radical species and free radical clearance mechanisms and anti-oxidant defence systems. Oxidative stress is one of the most important potential causes of age-related deterioration in neuronal function, and cumulative damage by free radicals may contribute to the late-life onset and progressive course of human neurodegenerative diseases such as ALS. There is particular interest in the role of oxidative stress in ALS because genetically determined abnormalities in the free radical defence system caused by mutations in Cu/Zn superoxide dismutase (SOD1) underlie one-fifth of cases of familial ALS, or approximately 2% of cases of ALS as a whole (Rosen et al., 1993; Radunovic and Leigh, 1996) (see Chapter 4).

SOD-1 is the cytosolic form of superoxide dismutase. Other forms include Mn-SOD, which is located within mitochondria, and extracellular SOD. SOD1 is a metalloenzyme comprising 153 amino acids with copper and zinc binding sites. It functions as a homodimer, with a copper ion in position at the base of its active channel. Copper is retained in the depths of the active channel by four histidine residues, and is an essential cofactor for the conversion of the superoxide anion to hydrogen peroxide (H_2O_2). The active site channel of normal SOD-1 may impose spatial constraints on the access of copper to reductants. The primary role of superoxide dismutase is to catalyze the dismutation of superoxide radicals to H_2O_2, which is then eliminated by the anti-oxidant enxymes glutathione peroxidase or catalase. Subsidiary activities of SOD1 include peroxidase activity resulting in the generation of hydroxyl radicals from H_2O_2 (Wiedau-Pazos et al., 1996), the production of nitronium species from peroxynitrite (Beckman et al., 1993), and the protection of the enzyme calcineurin from inactivation (Wang et al., 1996).

To date, more than 60 different mutations in the *SOD1* gene have been described in more than 250 ALS pedigrees, involving all five exons (Siddique et al., 1996; Shaw et al., 1998a) and rarely noncoding sequences (Shaw et al., 1997b). The majority are single base-pair exonic substitutions. The described mutations tend to affect the dimer stability or beta-barrel folding of the enzyme (Brown, 1995). SOD-1 activity assayed in red blood cells, in transformed lymphoblastoid cell lines, and in brain tissue from ALS cases is reduced to 30–70% of that in control samples. This may result from the lower stability and reduced half-life of the mutant protein (Borchelt et al., 1995). However, it may be misleading to correlate the SOD-1 activities measured in vitro directly with the SOD1 activity in motor neurons.

Some insights into potential mechanisms of motor neuron injury in the presence of *SOD1* mutations have been gained, though the precise sequence of cellular events has not yet been delineated. It has been established that normal human motor neurons have a high expression of SOD1 in both perikaryal and axonal compartments, compared to other groups of neurons in the CNS (Pardo et al., 1995; Shaw et al., 1997a). It has not yet been established with certainty whether a loss of function or a toxic gain of function of mutant SOD1, or both, is responsible for motor neuron injury, nor is it established whether all *SOD1* mutations have the same pathophysiological effects.

Loss of function hypothesis

The loss of function hypothesis postulates that motor neuron injury occurs by the direct effect of superoxide radicals inadequately scavenged by the mutant SOD1 protein. This hypothesis is lent some support by the following observations:

1 Mutant SOD-1 in *Drosophila* causes a dominant negative effect on the normal SOD1 protein (Phillips et al., 1995).
2 There are a large number of mutations in *SOD1* which lead to a reduction in cytosolic enzyme activity but are not predicted to produce similar structural changes in the protein (Siddique et al., 1996).

3 In organotypic spinal cord cultures and cultures of PC12 cells, reduction of SOD1 activity by pharmacological means or the application of anti-sense oligonucleotides triggers cell death by apoptosis (Troy and Shelanski, 1994; Rothstein et al., 1994a).

Nevertheless, loss of SOD1 activity is not sufficient to cause motor neuron disease, as not all *SOD1* mutations in ALS cause low activity; further, the *SOD1* knockout mouse does not develop an ALS phenotype. However, motor neurons in this mouse model are more susceptible to cell death following an insult such as axotomy (Reaume et al., 1996).

However, there is a compelling body of scientific evidence, including observations from *SOD1* transgenic mice, which favors the possibility that the mutant SOD1 protein is causing motor neuron injury by a toxic gain of function deleterious to these cells (Figure 3.4). Several hypotheses have been generated to explain this. Many of the missense mutations in *SOD1* have the potential to alter the active site of the SOD1 enzyme. X-ray crytallographic studies have shown that the active channel of the mutant SOD1 protein is slightly larger than that of the wild-type enzyme, thus allowing greater accessiblity or unshielding of the active copper site (Deng et al., 1993). Such changes could allow mutant SOD1 to react with additional substrates such as H_2O_2 and peroxynitrite, as well as its normal substrate of superoxide anions (Brown, 1995; Beckman et al., 1993).

Toxic gain of function hypothesis

Four main hypotheses have been put forward to explain the toxic gain of function of mutant SOD1.

Nitration of protein tyrosine residues

Under normal physiological conditions the superoxide anion can combine with nitric oxide to form peroxynitrite. This process may be enhanced as the activity of SOD1 decreases and the levels of intracellular superoxide increase. Normal or mutant SOD1 can catalyze nitration of tyrosine residues of proteins by accepting peroxynitrite as a substrate, which results in the formation of nitronium ions. The more open active site channel of the mutant SOD1 protein may enhance the access of peroxynitrite to the active site. Neurofilament proteins and neurotrophic factor (tyrosine kinase) receptors are proteins particularly susceptible to nitrotyrosine damage, and both are crucial for the normal function of motor neurons (Beckman et al., 1993).

Hyroxyl radical formation

Under certain conditions hydrogen peroxide can interact with copper in the active site of SOD1 to form hydroxyl radicals. Under normal circumstances the charge profile of the enzyme channel and the local rate of production of hydrogen peroxide preclude the formation of significant quantities of hydroxyl radicals. However, it is possible that SOD1 mutations might result in unshielding of the active copper site increasing the accessibility to hydrogen peroxide and/or may retard the egress of hydrogen peroxide, thereby augmenting

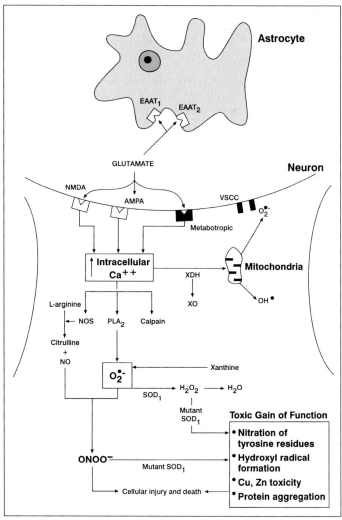

Fig. 3.4 Summary of the potential interactions between glutamate receptor activation, elevation of intracellular calcium, mitochondrial dysfunction and oxidative stress. These interacting mechanisms can potentially lead to an escalating cascade of cellular injury resulting in damage to critical subcellular organelles and proteins. Binding of glutamate to its cell surface receptors triggers an elevation of cytosolic calcium. This increase in intracellular free calcium activates a number of enzyme systems including nitric oxide synthase (NOS), which generates nitric oxide (NO) and phospholipase A_2 (PLA$_2$) which generates superoxide ($O_2^{\cdot-}$) radicals. Ca^{++} also converts xanthine dehydrogenase (XDH) to xanthine oxidase (XO), leading to the formation of $O_2^{\cdot-}$ from xanthine. Elevated Ca^{++} may also be toxic to mitochondria, resulting in release of OH· and $O_2^{\cdot-}$ radicals. Normal SOD1 converts $O_2^{\cdot-}$ to hydrogen peroxide (H_2O_2), which is further metabolized to H_2O by the action of the free radical scavenging enzymes glutathione peroxidase and catalase. Under normal phsiological conditions, NO may combine with $O_2^{\cdot-}$ to form peroxynitrite (ONOO$^-$). The four main hypotheses for the toxic gain of function in the presence of mutant SOD1 are nitration of tyrosine residues of proteins by derivatives of peroxynitrite, hydroxyl radical formation resulting from altered reactivity to H_2O_2 in the active channel of mutant SOD1, cellular toxicity resulting from the release of Cu^{++} and Zn^{++}, and aggregation of mutant protein

the formation of hydroxyl radicals. Hydroxyl radicals may react in situ with SOD1 itself, thereby inactivating the enzyme, or may diffuse out into the cytosol to interact with other targets.

Copper and zinc toxicity

Experiments in yeast and bacteria indicate that mutant SOD1 proteins do not bind metals normally. Elevated intracellular levels of copper and zinc may be directly toxic to neurons. Copper may participate in potentially harmful redox reactions and zinc may interact with glutamate receptors.

Protein aggregation

It has been suggested that mutant SOD1 protein may accumulate and form toxic intracellular aggregates. Some support is given to this hypothesis from recent observations in post-mortem material from ALS patients and from cellular models of *SOD1*-related familial ALS (Shibata et al., 1993; Durham et al., 1997).

Insights gained from *SOD1* transgenic mice

Three mutant transgenic *SOD1* mouse strains, G93A, G85R, and G37R, have been demonstrated to develop an ALS-like phenotype (Gurney et al., 1994; Ripps et al., 1995; Wong et al., 1995). Transgenic mice with wild-type human SOD1 expressed at similar levels do not develop motor neuron disease. The mutant *SOD1* mice develop progressive weakness and wasting affecting limb and bulbar muscles. The behavioral manifestations of the disease usually start between 3 and 8 months of age and animals then usually die within a few weeks. The spinal and brainstem lower motor neurons are primarily affected, but pathologic changes have also been shown in the corticospinal tract and sensory pathways (Dal Canto and Gurney, 1995). These mice are important animal models for ALS research, but it should be noted that there are important differences from human familial ALS.

- First, *SOD1* transgenic mice contain more copies of the mutant human *SOD1* gene than do human familial ALS patients.
- Second, the emergence of motor neuron disease in these mice requires several fold over-expression of mutant SOD1.
- Third, G93A and G37R transgenic mice develop a striking vacuolar pathology which has not been a recognized component of human ALS.

Therefore, a degree of caution must be exercised in extrapolating data from these transgenic mice to human ALS. Nevertheless, the mice provide an important tool for examining the progression of cellular events underlying motor neuron injury, for testing hypotheses relating to the mechanism of cell death, and for evaluating therapeutic agents.

Cellular pathology

The different mutations produce varying cellular pathology. The G93A and G37R mice tend to develop early changes of vacuolation in dendrites and axons of motor neurons, with reactive gliosis, followed by vacuolation of the perikarya and cell death. Prominent swelling and vacuolation of mitochondria and fragmentation of the Golgi apparatus are early features of the cellular pathology. The G93A mutant develops abnormal neurofilamentous accumulations akin to those present in human ALS. The G85R mutant develops early morphological changes within glia, with inclusions that are immunoreactive with antibodies to SOD1 and ubiquitin (Bruijn and Cleveland 1996; Bruijn et al., 1997). These changes are accompanied by reduced expression of the glutamate transporter protein GLT-1. It has been demonstrated that G93A mice expressing a low copy number of the transgene develop pathology most closely resembling the changes found in human ALS (Dal Canto and Gurney, 1994; Tu et al., 1996). In these mice there is motor neuron degeneration associated with neuronal and filamentous inclusions which show positive immunoreactivity for neurofilaments and ubiquitin, together with astrocytic inclusions. Kong and Xu (1998) showed in G93A mice that the onset of the disease involves a sharp decline in muscle strength and a transient explosive increase in vacuoles derived from degenerating mitochondria, but little motor neuron death. Most motor neurons did not die until the terminal stage of the disease, approximately 9 weeks after the behavioral features first became evident. The interpretation of these authors is that mutant SOD1 toxicity is mediated by damage to mitochondria in motor neurons and that this damage triggers the functional decline of motor neurons, heralding the onset of ALS. They suggest that the absence of motor neuron death in the early stages of the disease indicates that the majority of motor neurons could potentially be rescued after diagnosis.

Neurochemistry

Ferrante and colleagues (1997a, b) have demonstrated significant increases in the concentration of 3-nitrotyrosine, a marker of peroxynitrite-mediated nitration, in the spinal cord of mice with the G93A *SOD1* mutation. Malondialdehyde, a marker of lipid peroxidation, was increased in the cerebral cortex. Immunoreactivity for 3-nitrotyrosine and malondialdehyde alteration of proteins were increased throughout the G93A mice spinal cord, the changes being particularly impressive within motor neurons. Bruijn and co-workers (1996) showed that 3-nitrotyrosine levels were elevated two- to three-fold in the spinal cords of G37R mice, coincident with the earliest pathological changes, and remained elevated in spinal cord throughout the progressive course of the disease. These findings indicate that oxidative damage and increased nitration of protein residues are important aspects of the biochemical pathology of *SOD1* mutations.

Therapeutic effects

The SOD1 transgenic mice provide a very important tool to examine the clinical effects of neuroprotective strategies. The clinical and pathological similarities between familial SOD1-related and sporadic ALS suggest that some common pathophysiological mechanisms may apply. There is therefore the possibility that therapeutic approaches showing a positive effect in *SOD1* transgenic mice may also have relevance in patients with sporadic ALS. In the G37R transgenic mouse, the anti-oxidant vitamin E delays the onset of disease but does not extend survival, whereas the anti-glutamate agent riluzole extends survival but does not delay the onset of the disease (Gurney et al., 1996). These findings suggest that different mechanisms may be operating at different stages of motor neuron injury, with oxidative stress having an important role at an early stage and glutamate toxicity playing a role later in the pathophysiological cascade. Several recent experiments have been undertaken in which *SOD1* transgenic mice have been crossed with other transgenic strains, to explore the effects of alterations in the expression of other genes on the course of the murine motor neuron disease. Over expression of the anti-apoptotic protein Bcl-2 (Kostic et al., 1997) and expression of a dominant negative inhibitor of the interleukin-1-β-converting enzyme (Friedlander et al., 1997) retard progression of the disease and extend survival.

SOD1 mutations: insights from cellular models

Several in vitro models of familial ALS have been generated based on the expression of *SOD1* mutations in cultured neurons. Yim and co-workers (1997) overexpressed cDNAs for the G93A *SOD1* mutation and wild-type SOD1 in Sf9 insect cells, purified the proteins, and studied their capacity for catalyzing the dismutation of superoxide anions and for generating free radicals with H_2O_2 as a substrate. Both enzymes had identical dismutation activity. However, the free radical generating function of G93A SOD1 was enhanced relative to the wild-type enzyme, due to a small decrease in the value of the K_m for H_2O_2. In vitro studies from the laboratory of Bredesen and colleagues have shown that at least two of the described *SOD1* mutations can increase the rate of hydroxyl radical formation, probably due to increased availability of the copper at the active site of the enzyme to H_2O_2 (Wiedau-Pazos et al., 1996). This group also showed that, when expressed in a neuronal cell line, the mutant SOD1 protein led to an increase in cell death under conditions of oxidative stress produced by serum or growth factor withdrawal. In contrast, overexpression of wild-type SOD1 inhibited apoptotic cell death (Rabizadeh et al., 1995). Other groups have prepared primary cultures of dopaminergic neurons from *SOD1* transgenic mice (Mena et al., 1997) or have transfected cell lines with adenoviral constructs containing mutant or wild-type SOD1 (Ghadge et al., 1997). In these experimental paradigms mutant SOD1 also enhances apoptotic cell death, whereas normal SOD1 has a neuroprotective effect. Cell death in the presence of mutant SOD1 could be prevented by Cu chelators, glutathione, vitamin E, inhibitors of caspase enzymes and increased expression of the anti-apoptotic protein Bcl-2 (Ghadge et al., 1997).

In a motor neuron cell line (NSC34) stably transfected with wild-type or mutant SOD1, the expression of mutant SOD1 enhanced cell death induced by serum withdrawal. In addition, the presence of *SOD1* mutations led to abnormal accumulations of neurofilament proteins (Cookson et al., 1997). In vitro experiments have indicated that nitration of neurofilament proteins is catalyzed by mutant SOD1 (Crow et al., 1997a,b). These studies suggest that neurofilament proteins are one of the major targets affected by the oxidative stress induced by mutant SOD1.

Microinjection of mutant SOD1 expression constructs into primary neurons in culture enhances the naturally occurring cell death of motor neurons, but not of other neuronal types (Durham et al., 1997). In this experimental system the motor neurons also developed SOD1 immunoreactive inclusions.

Indices of oxidative stress in human familial and sporadic ALS
Familial ALS

To date, only a small number of cases of human ALS with defined *SOD1* mutations have undergone detailed postmortem neurochemical investigation, and relatively little information is available on the neurochemical pathology in this subgroup of patients. Ferrante and colleagues reported increased immunostaining for haemoxygenase-1 (a protein whose expression is increased in the presence of oxidative stress), malondialdehyde-modified protein (produced as a product of lipid peroxidation reactions), and 8-hydroxy-2'deoxyguanosine (an adduct formed by oxidative damage to DNA) in five cases of *SOD1*-linked familial ALS (Ferrante et al., 1997a, b). These neurochemical changes are remarkably similar to those described in *SOD1* transgenic mice discussed in an earlier section.

Sporadic ALS

In relation to sporadic ALS, several lines of evidence have emerged which suggest that oxidative stress may be operating as a contributory factor to motor neuron injury.

Cellular responses to oxidative stress   One study has investigated the sensitivity of fibroblasts cultured from patients with sporadic ALS (SALS) as well as familial ALS (FALS) to oxidative stress induced by exposure to H_2O_2, SIN-1 (3-morpholinosydranimine, an agent which induces the formation of both nitric oxide and superoxide radicals), and serum withdrawal (Aguirre et al., 1998). SALS and FALS fibroblasts were significantly more sensitive to SIN-1 than those of controls, whereas only FALS fibroblasts were more sensitive to H_2O_2. These results suggest that impaired cellular defence against oxidative stress may be important in the pathophysiology of sporadic as well as SOD1-related familial ALS.

Biochemical indices of oxidative damage   Studies from two different laboratories have shown that protein carbonyls, formed by oxidative modification of specific amino acid residues in proteins, are higher in the spinal cord (Shaw et al., 1995a, b) and frontal cortex (Bowling et al., 1993) of sporadic ALS patients than in normals or in neurological disease with similar agonal status. The spinal cord of sporadic ALS patients shows a higher concentration of 3-nitrotyrosine, a marker of peroxynitrite mediated protein damage, than in controls (Beal et al., 1997). Increased protein nitrosylation has also been demonstrated in residual motor neurons from sporadic ALS cases using immunohistochemistry (Abe et al., 1995; Beal et al., 1997). Ferrante et al. (1997a, b) reported an increase in biochemical indices of oxidative damage to proteins and DNA in the spinal cord and motor cortex of sporadic ALS cases. CSF levels of 4-hydroxynonenal, a lipid peroxidation product which is cytotoxic to neurons, are increased in sporadic ALS, as compared to other neurologic disease controls (Smith et al., 1998). This provides an important context to the postmortem studies discussed above, because it proves that markers of oxidative damage are present in life, earlier in the disease process.

Biochemical indices which may indicate an attempted compensatory response to oxidative stress   The level of selenium and the activity of the selenium-containing enzyme glutathione peroxidase are elevated in the spinal cord of ALS patients compared with controls (Ince et al., 1994). Glutathione peroxidase is a free radical scavenging enzyme which operates downstream from SOD1 with catalase, whose function is to catalyze the conversion of H_2O_2 produced by SOD1. A later study, however, reported that the activity of glutathione peroxidase was reduced in the cortex of ALS patients (Przedborski et al., 1996). SOD1 mRNA has been shown to be increased in individual surviving motor neurons from cases of sporadic ALS (Bergeron et al., 1994). Immunohistochemical studies have shown increased expression of SOD1, Mn SOD, and catalase, predominantly in glia, in the vicinity of the corticospinal tracts and/or neuropil of the ventral horn in sporadic ALS (Shaw et al., 1997a, b). Increased glial expression of metallothionein has also been shown in the spinal cord of ALS patients (Sillevis Smitt et al., 1994). Metallothioneins are of interest in relation to cellular defence against oxidative stress, as they function as metal binding proteins with free radical scavenging capabilities.

Derangement of intracellular calcium homeostasis

Calcium plays a fundamental role in many normal cellular processes, including neuronal excitability and regulation of intracellular second messenger systems. Following influx into the cytosol, calcium binds to calmodulin and stimulates the activity of a variety of enzymes including calcium-calmodulin kinases and calcium-sensitive adenylate cyclases. These enzymes transduce the calcium signal and effect short-term biological responses such as modification of synaptic proteins and long-lasting neuronal responses that require changes in gene expression. In addition to changes in the level of intracellular calcium, the route of calcium entry and its intracellular localisation are important in determining the physiological responses.

The concentration of intracellular free calcium is tightly controlled in most neurons at approximately 100 nm (Siesjo, 1988). This is about four orders of magnitude less than the extracellular level. A number of subcellular systems are important in the control of intracellular calcium homeostasis, including:

- membrane Ca^{++} channels that allow Ca^{++} to move down its concentration gradient into the cytoplasm;
- plasma membrane Na^+/Ca^{++} exchangers;

▦ ATP-dependent Ca++ pumps;
▦ sequestration in cytoplasmic organelles including the endoplasmic reticulum and mitochondria;
▦ calcium-binding proteins such as parvalbumin, calbindin D28k, and calretinin.

Within the nervous system, some differences in Ca++ homeostatic systems are clearly cell specific.

Intracellular calcium homeostasis is inextricably linked with other potential mechanisms underlying degeneration of motor neurons described in this chapter, including glutamatergic toxicity, oxidative stress, and mitochondrial dysfunction. Activation of cell surface glutamate receptors is a major route for calcium entry into neurons. Both NMDA receptors and AMPA receptors lacking the GluR2 subunit have calcium-permeable ion channels. In addition, depolarization of a neuron by activation of glutamate receptors may lead to a secondary influx of calcium resulting from activation of voltage-gated calcium channels. Sustained elevation of intracellular calcium resulting from glutamate receptor activation can eventually lead to neuronal injury due to excessive activation of several enzyme cascades and the formation of free radicals resulting in oxidative stress (Siesjo, 1994). The enzymes activated by intracellular calcium include lipases, proteases, protein kinases/phosphatases, calmodulin-dependent enzymes and endonucleases (Choi, 1990, 1994). Activation of lipases (e.g. phospholipase A_2) leads to membrane degradation and the production of free radicals via the arachidonic acid cascade. Activation of proteases (e.g. the calpains) can result in cleavage of cytoskeletal proteins. Stimulation of protein kinases (e.g. protein kinase C) and phosphatases can lead to modulation of cell surface receptors and channels and to alterations in gene expression (Choi, 1994; Brorson et al., 1995). Activation of endonuclease results in degradation of genomic DNA. Inhibitors of calpains, protein kinase C, and endonucleases have all been found to protect neurons in culture from glutamate-mediated toxicity (Brorson et al., 1995; Krieger et al., 1996; Rothstein and Kuncl, 1995).

The production of intracellular free radicals can lead to several destructive processes, including lipid peroxidation and oxidative damage to proteins and DNA. Intracellular calcium can generate free radical production by:

1 The metabolism of arachidonic acid by lipoxygenases and cycloxygenases.
2 The activation of xanthine oxidase.
3 Activation of nitric oxide synthase and the release of nitric oxide (Siesjo, 1994).

Mitochondria act as an important intracellular store for calcium. It has been suggested that the permeability transition pore in the mitochondrial membrane may act as a calcium release channel involved in calcium homeostasis in the cell (Bernardi, 1996; Bernardi and Petronilli, 1996).

The possibility that spinal motor neurons may be particularly vulnerable to calcium-mediated injury is suggested by the observations that this cell population appears to lack the expression of the Ca++ buffering proteins parvalbumin and calbindin D28K (Ince et al., 1993), while expressing abundant calpain

II, a calcium-activated proteolytic enzyme (Li et al., 1996). Motor neuron groups such as the oculomotor neurons that are less vulnerable to pathology in ALS do express parvalbumin. In addition, as discussed above, the expression of calcium-permeable AMPA receptors by human motor neurons (Williams et al., 1997) may be a further factor contributing to the vulnerability of this cell group to calcium-mediated toxic processes.

Siklos et al. (1996) investigated motor axon terminals in muscle biopsies from patients with ALS and found increased calcium, increased mitochondrial volume, and increased numbers of synaptic vesicles. In a subsequent study the same group demonstrated that motor neurons of transgenic mice with a G93A *SOD1* mutation exhibit alterations in intracellular calcium, using the oxalate–pyroantimonate technique and ultrastructural examination (Siklos et al., 1998). The cell bodies and proximal dendrites of spinal motor neurons contained small vacuoles filled with calcium, in mice aged 60 days. In contrast, oculomotor neurons, (which, unlike spinal motor neurons, contain the calcium-binding protein parvalbumin) showed only minimal evidence of degeneration, no vacuolation, and no increased calcium or altered calcium distribution. The authors concluded that the free radical-mediated stress induced by mutant SOD1 appeared to induce deleterious changes in intracellular calcium distribution in motor neuron populations lacking calbindin D28K and/or parvalbumin, whereas motor neurons possessing these calcium-binding proteins were more resistant to the stress.

Candidate cellular targets for injury in motor neuron degeneration in ALS
Glial proteins involved in the regulation of the glutamate neurotransmitter system

Glutamine synthetase (GS) is a glial enzyme which is a key component of the glutamine–glutamate cycle, essential for the recycling of neurotransmitter glutamate. GS converts glutamate to glutamine, which is then transported back to the neuronal terminal where it is converted back to glutamate (Laake et al., 1995). A decrease in GS activity results in an increase in extracellular glutamate and a decrease in neuronal glutamate (Schousboe et al., 1993), neurochemical alterations similar to those described in ALS. However, GS activity is normal in ALS in motor cortex (Rothstein and Kuncl, reviewed in Rothstein, 1996).

As discussed in a previous section, the astrocytic glutamate transporter proteins EAAT1 and EAAT2 are essential for the removal of glutamate from the synaptic cleft and for termination of its excitatory signal. In vitro, both GS and EAAT2 have been shown to be highly susceptible to oxidative damage (Volterra et al., 1994; Schor, 1988). Both of these proteins are therefore candidate targets for damage in ALS, and warrant further investigation.

Neurofilament proteins

Neurofilament proteins especially deserve description, as they form a major component of the cytoskeleton of neurons and have significant roles in the maintenance of cell shape and axonal calibre as well as in axonal transport. Neurofilaments are the most abundant structural proteins in large cells with long axons, like motor neurons. Neurofilaments are composed of three subunit polypeptides: neurofilament light, NF-L (MW 68kDa); neurofilament medium, NF-M (MW 150kDa); and neurofilament heavy, NF-H (MW 200kDa), assembled in a 6:2:1 ratio to form macromolecular filaments (Nixon and Shea, 1992) (Figure 3.5). Each neurofilament subunit consists of conserved head and rod domains, and a more variable acidic tail domain. The rod domains are principally composed of α-helices, which wrap around each other to form a superhelix of parallel coiled coils (Lupas, 1996). The head domain is important for the lateral interactions between neurofilaments (Heins et al., 1993). The assembly of neurofilaments involves many complex interactions between subunits, stabilized by hydrophobic interactions which often involve tyrosine residues. The smallest protein (NF-L) makes up the core of the neurofilament, while the two larger proteins (NF-M and NF-H) are arranged around this core and contribute to the projections or side arms radiating from the filament. Neurofilament subunits are assembled in the motor neuron perikaryon and are transported down the axon by slow axonal transport at a rate of 1 mm per day. Some phosphorylation of neurofilaments occurs within the cell body, and, under normal circumstances, phosphorylation progressively increases as the neurofilament proteins are transported down the axon.

Neurofilament proteins are of considerable interest in ALS as potential cellular targets for injury for several reasons. The abnormal assembly and accumulation of neurofilaments in the perikaryon and proximal axons of motor

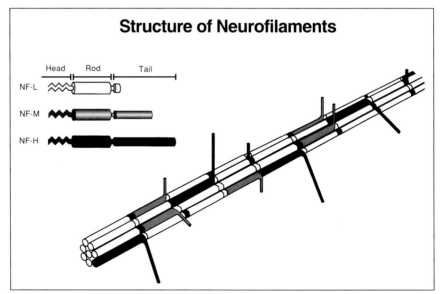

Fig. 3.5 Structure of neurofilaments. Three neurofilament polypeptides NF-L, NF-M and NF-H assemble to form macromolecular filaments. Each neurofilament subunit consists of conserved head and rod domains and a more variable acidic tail domain. The smallest protein (NF-L) makes up the core of the neurofilament, while the two larger proteins (NF-M and NF-H) are arranged around this core and contribute to the projections or side arms radiating from the filament

neurons is a characteristic feature of the pathology of ALS (Hirano, 1991). It is unclear whether the neurofilament accumulations in proximal axons may cause impaired axonal transport or may arise secondarily to a block in axonal transport. Increased phosphorylation of neurofilaments within the motor neuron cell body can be observed following several types of cellular insult. Consensus has not been reached as to whether phosphorylated neurofilaments are increased in cell bodies of surviving motor neurons in ALS: some studies have reported an increase in the perikaryal expression of phosphorylated neurofilaments (Sobue et al., 1990; Manetto et al., 1988; Munoz et al., 1988), but others have failed to replicate this observation (Leigh et al., 1989). Ubiquitinated inclusions with compact or Lewy body-like morphology in surviving motor neurons in ALS may show immunoreactivity for neurofilament epitopes (Murayama 1989; Ince et al., 1998b). In some cases of SOD1-related familial ALS, large argyrophilic hyaline conglomerate inclusions have been observed in the cell bodies and axons of motor neurons (Ince et al., 1998b; Rouleau et al., 1996). These show strong immunoreactivity with antibodies to both phosphorylated and nonphosphorylated neurofilaments (Figure 3.6).

The importance of neurofilaments in the normal health of motor neurons is underscored by the finding that occasional cases of sporadic ALS have deletions or insertions in the KSP repeat region of the *NF-H* gene (Figlewicz et al., 1994; Tomkins et al., 1998). In addition, motor neuron pathological changes develop in transgenic mice overexpressing NF-L or NF-H subunits (Xu et al., 1993; Cote et al., 1993) or in mice expressing mutations in the *NF-L* gene (Lee et al., 1994). These in vivo models demonstrate that disruption of neurofilament assembly can injure motor neurons relatively selectively.

Transgenic mice that carry mutations in the human *SOD1* gene also show neuropathological changes affecting neurofilament organization. The G93A mutant transgenic mouse develops spheroids within motor neurons which contain both phosphorylated and nonphosphorylated neurofilaments (Tu et al., 1996). These neurofilament accumulations may account for the reduction in

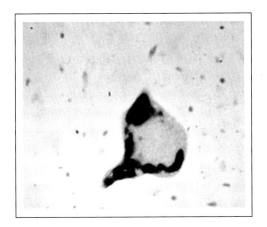

Fig. 3.6 Lumbar motor neuron from a patient with an I113T SOD1 mutation showing extensive hyaline conglomerate inclusions. These are stained by antibodies to both phosphorylated and nonphosphorylated neurofilament epitopes

neurofilament protein and the rate of transport seen in the ventral root axons of G93A transgenic mice (Zhang et al., 1997).

In neuronal cell culture models of oxidative stress, neurofilament proteins appear to show differential vulnerability to free radical damage (Cookson et al., 1996). Motor neuron cell lines transfected with mutant *SOD1* also show accumulations of neurofilament proteins which are not seen in the presence of normal *SOD1* (Cookson et al., 1997). As described above, one of the major hypotheses for the toxic gain of function associated with *SOD1* mutations is that altered substrate affinity of the active site of the mutant enzyme may lead to nitration of tyrosine residues of susceptible proteins, as a result of generation of nitronium residues from peroxynitrite (Beckman et al., 1993). It has been shown that the tyrosine residues in the rod and tail domains of NF-L are more susceptible to SOD1-catalyzed nitration than other proteins in the CNS (Crow et al., 1997a). Other factors that may contribute to the vulnerability of neurofilament proteins to oxidative stress include their long half-lives and their high content of lysine, an amino acid residue susceptible to oxidative modification.

Mitochondria

It is now widely accepted that glutamate receptor activation, free radical damage, and mitochondrial energy metabolism are interconnected pathways central to the pathogenesis of cell death in the nervous system. These mechanisms are linked through the intracellular actions of calcium.

Mitochondria are both producers and targets of reactive oxygen species. They are the most important source for the intracellular generation of free radicals within neurons. Both superoxide radicals and hydrogen peroxide are generated within mitochondria, accounting for up to 4% of oxygen metabolism under resting conditions (Boveris and Chance, 1973). It has been demonstrated that mitochondrial production of free radicals increases both in isolated mitochondria under conditions of a calcium load equivalent to glutamate receptor activation (Dykens, 1994) and in cultured neurons exposed to glutamate (Dugan et al., 1994). Conversely, mitochondria themselves are particularly susceptible to free radical damage at both protein and DNA levels (DiMonte et al., 1993; Bowling and Beal, 1995), and free radicals are known to inhibit the activities of specific mitochondrial enzymes (Zhang et al., 1990). The most sensitive mitochondrial proteins appear to be NADH dehydrogenase, ATPase, and succinate dehydrogenase.

Age-related changes in mitochondrial function have been suggested as an important factor contributing to late-onset neurodegenerative diseases. There is evidence for age-related deterioration in mitochondrial function, for accumulation of mutations in mitochondrial DNA, and for a decline in brain glucose metabolism in human brain. Mitochondria contain five enzyme complexes comprising the electron transport chain responsible for the synthesis of ATP. In nonhuman primates, a decline in the activities of mitochondrial respiratory chain complexes I and IV has been demonstrated during normal neuronal aging (Beal et al., 1993; Richter, 1995) and similar changes have been reported in human muscle (Boffoli et al., 1994). This defect in energy metabolism may exert no effect until the neuron falls to below a critical threshold of energy production, when it may become susceptible to secondary excito-toxicity and other injurious processes (Meccoci et al., 1993).

A significant factor contibuting to the age-related decline in mitochondrial function is the effect of accumulating mutations in the mitochondrial genome (Linnane et al., 1989). Mitochondrial DNA consists of 13 genes encoding sub-units of the electron transport chain and is particularly vulnerable to oxida-tive damage. Several factors may contribute to this vulnerability, including the very low ratio of noncoding to coding sequences compared with nuclear DNA, the proximity to the major intracellular source of free radical production, together with minimal provision of DNA repair mechanisms and the absence of protective histones in the vicinity of mitochondrial DNA. The accumula-tion of mitochondrial DNA mutations is particularly prominent in post-mitotic tissues such as the CNS, and is demonstrable as higher levels of 8-OH-2-deoxyguanosine in mitochondrial than in nuclear DNA (Richter et al., 1988).

The possibility that mitochondrial dysfunction may contribute to motor neuron injury in ALS has not yet been systematically studied. However, some evidence is emerging to indicate that mitochondrial dysfunction may be an important problem in this disease. Cytochrome c oxidase activity in post-mortem spinal cord is reportedly decreased in ALS (Fujita et al., 1996). In frontal cortex from cases of familial ALS, the complex 1 component of the electron transport chain was altered (Bowling et al., 1993). A microdeletion in subunit 1 of cytochrome oxidase C has been described in one patient with an ALS phenotype (Comi et al., 1998). Evidence of mitochondrial dysfunction may also be seen in lymphocytes from ALS patients (Curti et al., 1996). Finally, in reports of pathological changes in *SOD1* transgenic mice, it has been empha-sized that vacuolar distortion of mitochondria occurs at an early stage in the cascade of motor neuron injury, before the appearance of behavioral signs of motor dysfunction (Wong et al., 1995, Chiu et al., 1995, Kong and Xu, 1998).

Given these clues, the possibility that mitochondrial dysfunction may be important in the pathway of motor neuron degeneration needs to be more sys-tematically examined. Impetus was added to this line of inquiry by the find-ing that coenzyme Q_{10} (an essential cofactor of the electron transport chain and a potent free radical scavenger in mitochondrial membranes), and crea-tine monohydrate (a carrier of high energy phosphate across the mitochondr-ial membrane) both slightly prolonged lifespan in the transgenic mouse model of familial ALS (Matthews et al., 1998; Klivenyi et al., 1999).

Conclusions

Insights are beginning to emerge in relation to the normal neurochemistry and molecular phenotype of human motor neurons, which may help to account for the vulnerability of this cell group to the neurodegenerative process in ALS. We are also beginning to identify the potentially important subcellular targets that are preferetially injured in the cell death process.

Genetic factors are clearly important in the pathogenesis of ALS. However, much work remains to be done to identify the genetic abnormalities underlying

80% of cases of familial ALS and to determine more clearly whether genetic factors, in conjunction perhaps with environmental stresses, may be important in the etiology of sporadic ALS.

A large body of circumstantial evidence now indicates that an imbalance between excitatory/glutamatergic and inhibitory neurotransmission may contribute to motor neuron injury in ALS. Even if this imbalance is secondary to another primary pathogenetic process, modulation of the glutamate neurotransmitter system still represents an important target for therapeutic intervention in the cell death cascade.

There is now compelling evidence that oxidative stress may play a role in motor neuron injury in both familial SOD1-related and the sporadic form of ALS. The discovery of mutations in the *SOD1* gene in a proportion of cases of familial ALS has allowed the development of cellular and animal models of the disease. These models can be expected in the future to make a major contribution to our understanding of the sequential molecular events underlying motor neuron injury and death, and to generate more effective neuroprotective strategies for the benefit of patients suffering from ALS.

Acknowledgments

The authors are grateful for the continued support of their work on motor neuron diseases by the Wellcome Trust, the Medical Research Council, the Scottish Motor Neuron Disease Association (PJS); the Cal Ripken/Lou Gehrig Fund for Neuromuscular Disease, the Dino and Wendy Fabbri Fund for Neuromuscular Research, the Gail Rupertus Fund for Neuromuscular Research, the National Institute of Neurological Disorders and Stroke, and the Muscular Dystrophy Association of America (RWK).

References

Abe K, Pan LH, Watanabe M, Kato T, Itoyama Y (1995) Induction of nitrotyrosine-like immunoreactivity in the lower motor neuron of amyotrophic lateral sclerosis. Neurosci Lett 199: 152–154.

Aguirre T, Van den Bosch L, Goetschalckx K et al. (1998) Increased sensitivity of fibroblasts from amyotrophic lateral sclerosis patients to oxidative stress. Ann Neurol 43: 452–457.

Al-Chalabi A, Enayat ZE, Bakker MC et al. (1996) Association of apolipoprotein E ε4 allele with bulbar onset motor neuron disease. Lancet 347: 159–160.

Aoki M, Lin CLG, Rothstein JD et al. (1998) Mutations in the glutamate transporter EAAT2 gene do not cause abnormal EAAT2 transcripts in amyotrophic lateral sclerosis. Ann Neurol 43: 645–653.

Appel SH, Glenn Smith R, Alexianu M, Engelhardt J, Stefani E (1995) Autoimmunity as an etiological factor in sporadic amyotrophic lateral sclerosis. Adv Neurol 68: 47–57.

Arriza JL, Eliasof S, Kavanaugh MP, Amara SG (1997) Excitatory amino acid transporter 5, a retinal glutamate transporter coupled to a chloride conductance. Proc Natl Acad Sci USA 94: 4155–4160.

Baimbridge KG, Celio MR, Rogers SH (1992) Calcium binding proteins in the nervous system. Trends Neurosci 15: 303–308.

Beal MF (1993) Role of excitotoxicity in human neurological disease. Curr Opin Neurobiol 2: 657–662.

Beal MF, Hyman BT, Koroshetz W (1993) Do defects in mitochondrial energy metabolism underlie the pathology of neurodegenerative diseases. Trends Neurol Sci 16: 125–131.

Beal MF, Ferrante RJ, Browne SE, Matthews RT, Kowall NW, Brown RB (1997) Increased 3-nitrotyrosine in both sporadic and familial amyotrophic lateral sclerosis. Ann Neurol 42: 646–654.

Beckman JS, Carson M, Smith CD, Koppenol WH (1993) ALS, SOD and peroxynitrite. Nature 364: 584.

Bensimon G, Lacomblez L, Meininger V et al. (1994) A controlled trial of riluzole in amyotrophic lateral sclerosis. New Engl J Med 330: 585–591.

Bergeron C, Muntasser S, Somerville MJ, Weyer L, Percy ME (1994) Copper/zinc superoxide dismutase mRNA levels are increased in sporadic amyotrophic lateral sclerosis motorneurons. Brain Res 659: 272–276.

Bernardi P (1996) The permeability transition pore. Control points of a cyclosporin A – sensitive mitochondrial channel involved in cell death. Biocim Biophys Acta 1275: 5–9.

Bernardi P, Petronilli V (1996) The permeability transition pore as a mitochondrial calcium release channel: a critical appraisal. J Bioenerg Biomen 28: 131–138.

Bettler B, Mulle C (1995) Review: Neurotransmitter Receptors II: AMPA and kainate receptors. Neuropharmacology 34: 123–139.

Boffoli D, Scacco SC, Vergari R et al. (1994) Decline with age of the respiratory chain activity in human skeletal muscle. Biochim Biophys Acta 1226: 73–82.

Bondy SC, Lee DK (1993) Oxidative stress induced by glutamate receptor agonists. Brain Res 610: 229–233.

Borchelt DR, Guarnieri M, Wong PC et al. (1995) Superoxide dismutase 1 subunits with mutations linked to familial amyotrophic lateral sclerosis do not affect wild-type subunit function. J Biol Chem 270(7): 3234–3238.

Boveris A, Chance B (1973) The mitochondrial generation of hydrogen peroxide. Biochem J 134: 707–716.

Bowling AC, Beal MF (1995) Bioenergetic and oxidative stress in neurodegenerative diseases. Life Sci 56(14): 1151–1171.

Bowling AC, Schulz JB, Brown RH, Beal MF (1993) Superoxide dismutase activity, oxidative damage and mitochondrial energy metabolism in familial and sporadic amyotrophic lateral sclerosis. J Neurochem 61: 2322–2325.

Bristol LA, Rothstein JD (1996) Glutamate transporter gene expression in amyotrophic lateral sclerosis motor cortex. Ann Neurol 39: 676–679.

Brorson JR, Manzolillo PA, Gibbons SJ, Miller RJ (1995) AMPA receptor desensitization predicts the selective vulnerability of cerebellar Purkinje cells to excitotoxicity. J Neurosci 15(6): 4515–4524.

Brorson JR, Marcuccilli CJ, Miller RJ (1995) Delayed antagonism of calpain reduces excitotoxicity in cultured neurons. Stroke 26(7): 1259–1266.

Brown RHJ (1995) Amyotrophic lateral sclerosis: recent insights from genetics and transgenic mice. Cell 80: 687–692.

Bruijn LI, Cleveland DW (1996) Mechanisms of selective motor neuron death in ALS: insights from transgenic mouse models of motor neuron disease. Neuropathol Appl Neurobiol 22: 373–387.

Bruijn LI, Becher MW, Lee MK et al. (1997) ALS-linked SOD1 mutant G85R mediates damage to astrocytes and promotes rapidly progressive disease with SOD1 containing inclusions. Neuron 18: 327–338.

Burke RE (1990) Spinal cord: central horn. In: Shepherd GM (ed.) The Synaptic Organisation of the Brain. Oxford University Press: New York, pp. 88–132.

Burnashev N, Monyer H, Seeburg PH, Sakmann B (1992) Divalent ion permeability of AMPA receptor channels is dominated by the edited form of a single subunit. Neuron 8: 189–198.

Burnashev N, Zhou Z, Neher E, Sakmann B (1995) Fractional calcium currents through recombinant GluR channels of the NMDA, AMPA and kainate receptor subtypes. J Physiol 485(2): 403–418.

Canton T, Pratt J, Stutzmann JM, Imperato A, Boireau A (1998) Glutamate uptake is decreased tardively in the spinal cord of FALS mice. NeuroReport 9: 775–778.

Chari G, Shaw PJ, Sahgal A (1996) Non-verbal visual attention, but not recognition memory or learning processes are impaired in motor neuron disease. Neuropsychologica 34: 377–385.

Chinnery RM, Shaw PJ, Ince PG, Johnson M (1993) Autoradiographic distribution of binding sites for the non-NMDA receptor antagonist [3H]CNQX in human motor cortex, brainstem and spinal cord. Brain Res 630: 75–81.

Chiu AY, Zhai P, Dal Canto MC et al. (1995) Age-dependent penetrance of disease in a transgenic mouse model of familial amyotrophic lateral sclerosis. Mol Cell Neurosci 6: 349–362.

Choi DW (1987) Ionic dependence of glutamate neurotoxicity in cortical cell culture. J Neurosci 7: 369–379.

Choi DW (1990) Methods for antagonising glutamate neurotoxicity. Cerebrovasc Brain Metab Rev 2: 105–147.

Choi DW (1994) Calcium and excitotoxic neuronal injury. Ann NY Acad Sci 747: 162–171.

Comi GP, Bordoni A, Salani S et al. (1998) Cytochrome c oxidase subunit 1 microdeletion in a patient with motor neuron disease. Ann Neurol 43: 110–116.

Cookson MR, Thatcher NM, Ince PG, Shaw PJ (1996) Selective loss of neurofilament proteins after exposure of differentiated IMR-32 neuroblastoma cells to oxidative stress. Brain Res 738: 162–166.

Cookson MR, Eggett CJ, Chinnery RM et al. (1997) Cu/Zn superoxide dismutase mutations affect neurofilament metabolism in the NSC34 motor neuron cell line. Proceedings of the 8th International Symposium on ALS/MND.

Cote F, Collard JF, Julien JP (1993) Progressive neuropathy in transgenic mice expressing the human neurofilament heavy gene: a mouse model of amyotrophic lateral sclerosis. Cell 73: 35–46.

Couratier P, Hugon J, Sindou P, Vallat JM, Dumas M (1993) Cell culture evidence for neuron degeneration in amyotrophic lateral sclerosis being linked to AMPA/kainate receptors. Lancet 341: 265–268.

Coyle JT, Puttfarcken P (1993) Oxidative stress, glutamate and neurodegenerative disorders. Science 262: 689–695.

Crow JP, Sampson JB, Zhuang Y, Thompson JA, Beckman JS (1997a) Decreased zinc affinity of amyotrophic lateral sclerosis-associated superoxide dismutase mutants leads to enhanced catalysis of tyrosine nitration by peroxynitrite. J Neurochem 69: 1936–1944.

Crow JP, Ye YZ, Strong M, Kirk M, Barnes S, Beckman JS (1997b) Superoxide dismutase catalyzes nitration of tyrosines by peroxynitrite in the rod and head domains of neurofilament-L. J Neurochem 69: 1945–1953.

Curti D, AM, Facchetti G et al. (1996) Amyotrophic lateral sclerosis: oxidative energy metabolism and calcium homeostasis in peripheral blood lymphocytes. Neurology 47: 1060–1064.

Dal Canto MC, Gurney ME (1994) Development of central nervous system pathology in a murine transgenic model of human amyotrophic lateral sclerosis. Am J Pathol 145(6): 1271–1279.

Dal Canto MC, Gurney ME (1995) Neuropathological changes in two lines of mice carrying a transgene for mutant human Cu, Zn SOD and in mice expressing wild type human SOD: a model of familial amyotrophic lateral sclerosis (FALS). Brain Res 676: 24–40.

Danbolt NC, Storm-Mathisen J, Kanner BI (1992) A Na+-K coupled L-glutamate transporter purified from rat brain is localized in glial cell processes. Neuroscience 51: 295.

Day NC, Williams TL, Ince PG, Kamboj RK, Lodge D, Shaw PJ (1995) Distribution of AMPA-selective glutamate receptor subunits in the human hippocampus and cerebellum. Mol Brain Res 31: 17–32.

Debono MW, Canton T, Pradier L, Doble A, Blanchard JC (1993) Effects of riluzole on electrophysiological responses mediated by rat kainate and NMDA receptors expressed in xenopus oocytes. Eur J Pharmacol 235: 283–287.

Deng HX, Hentati A, Tainer J et al. (1993) Amyotrophic lateral sclerosis and structural defects in Cu/Zn superoxide dismutase. Science 261: 1047–1051.

Di Monte DA, Sandy MS, DeLanney LE et al. (1993) Age-dependent changes in mitochondrial energy metabolism in striatum and cerebellum of monkey brain. Neurodegeneration 2: 93–99.

Doble A, Hubert JP, Blanchard JC (1992) Pertussis toxin pretreatment abolishes the inhibitory effect of riluzole and carbachol on D-[³H] aspartate release from cultured cerebellar granule cells. Neurosci Lett 140: 251–254.

Dugan LL, Sensi SL, Canzoniero LMT et al. (1994) Imaging of mitochondrial oxygen radical production in cortical neurons exposed to NMDA. Soc Neurosci Abstr 19: 21.

Durham HD, Roy J, Dong L, Figlewicz DA (1997) Aggregation of mutant Cu/Zn superoxide dismutase proteins in a culture model of ALS. J Neuropath Exp Neurol 56: 523–530.

Dykens JA (1994) Isolated cerebral and cerebellar mitochondria produce free radicals when exposed to elevated Ca++ and Na+: implications for neurodegeneration. J Neurochem 63: 584–591.

Eisen A, Pant B, Stewart H (1993) Cortical excitability in amyotrophic lateral sclerosis: a clue to pathogenesis. Can J Neurol Sci 20: 11–16.

Estevez AG, Stutzmann J-M, Barbeito L (1995) Protective effect of riluzole on excitatory amino acid-mediated neurotoxicity in motoneuron-enriched cultures. Eur J Pharmacol 280: 47–53.

Fairman WA, Vandenberg RJ, Arriza JL, Kavanaugh MP, Amara SG (1995) An excitatory amino-acid transporter with properties of a ligand-gated chloride channel. Nature 375: 599–603.

Ferrante RJ, Browne SE, Shinobu LA et al. (1997a) Evidence of increased oxidative damage in both sporadic and familial amyotrophic lateral sclerosis. J Neurochem 69: 2064–2074.

Ferrante RJ, Shinobu LA, Schulz JB et al. (1997b) Increased 3-nitrotyrosine and oxidative damage in mice with a human copper/zinc superoxide dismutase mutation. Ann Neurol 42: 326–334.

Ferraro TN, Hare TA (1985) Free and conjugated amino acids in human CSF: influence of age and sex. Brain Res 338: 53–60.

Figlewicz DA, Rouleau GA, Krizus A, Julien JP (1994) Variants of the heavy neurofilament subunit are associated with the development of amyotrophic lateral sclerosis. Hum Mol Genet 3: 1757–1761.

Flowers JM, Powell JF, Leigh PN, Andersen P, Shaw CE (2001) Intron 7 retention and exon 9 skipping EAAT2 mRNA variants are not associated with amyotrophic lateral sclerosis. Ann Neurol 49: 643–649.

Fray AE, Ince PG, Banner SJ et al. (1998) The expression of the glial glutamate transporter protein EAAT2 in motor neuron disease: an immunocytochemical study. Eur J Neurosci 10: 2481–2489.

Friedlander RM, Brown RH, Gagliardini V, Wang J, Yuan J (1997) Inhibition of ICE slows ALS in mice. Nature 388: 31.

Fujita K, Yamauchi M, Shibayama K, Ando M, Honda M, Nagata Y (1996) Decreased cytochrome c oxidase activity but unchanged superoxide dismutase and glutathione peroxidase activities in the spinal cord of patients with amyotrophic lateral sclerosis. J Neurosci Res 45: 276–281.

Ghadge GD, Lee JP, Bindokas VP et al. (1997) Mutant superoxide dismutase-1-linked familial amyotrophic lateral sclerosis: molecular mechanisms of neuronal death and protection. J Neurosci 17: 8756–8766.

Girdlestone DA, Dupuy A, Roy-Contancin L, Escande D (1989) Riluzole antagonists excitatory amino acid evoked firing in rat facial motoneurons. Br J Pharmacol 97: 583P.

Gurney ME, Pu H, Chiu AY (1994) Motor neuron degeneration in mice that express a human Cu/Zn superoxide dismutase mutation. Science 264: 1772–1775.

Gurney ME, Cutting FB, Zhai P et al. (1996) Benefit of vitamin E, riluzole and gabapentin in a transgenic model of familial amyotrophic lateral sclerosis. Ann Neurol 39: 147–158.

Hattori T (1984) Negative symptoms and signs of amyotrophic lateral sclerosis: disturbance of micturition. Rinsho Sinkeigaku 24: 1254–1256.

Haugeto O, Ullensuang K, Levy LM et al. (1996) Brain glutamate transporters form homomultimers. J Biol Chem 271: 27715–27722.

Hebert T, Drapeau P, Pradier L, R.J.D (1994) Block of the rat brain 1A sodium channel subunit by the neuroprotective drug riluzole. Mol Pharmacol 45: 1055–1060.

Heins S, Wong PC, Muller S, Goldie K, Cleveland DW, Aebi U (1993) The rod domain of NF-L determines neurofilament architecture, whereas the end domains specify filament assembly and network formation. J Cell Biol 123: 1517–1533.

Hentati A, Bejaoui K, Pericak-Vance M et al. (1994) Linkage of recessive familial amyotrophic lateral sclerosis to chromosome 2q33-q35. Nature Genet 7: 425–427.

Hirano A (1991) Cytopathology of amyotrophic lateral sclerosis. Adv Neurol 56: 91–101.

Hollmann M, Heinemann S (1994) Cloned glutamate receptors. Annu Rev Neurosci 17: 31–108.

Honig LS, Gong Y-H, Bigio EH, Elliott JL (1999) Glutamate transporter EAAT-2 splice variants are not specific to ALS, but are present in normal and Alzheimer disease brains. Neurology 52 (suppl 2): 166–167.

Hubert JP, Delumeau JC, Glowinski J, Premont J, Doble A (1994) Antagonism by riluzone of entry of calcium evoked by NMDA and veratridine in rat cultured granule cells: evidence for a dual mechanism of action. Br J Pharmacol 113: 261–267.

Hugon J, Vallat JM (1990) Abnormal distribution of phosphorylated neurofilaments in neuronal degeneration induced by kainic acid. Neurosci Lett 119: 45–48.

Hume RI, Dingledine R, Heinemann S (1991) Identification of a site in glutamate receptor subunits that controls calcium permeability. Science 253: 1028–1031.

Ince PG, Stout N, Shaw PJ et al. (1993) Paravalbumin and calbindin D-28k in the human motor system and in motor neuron disease. Neuropathol Appl Neurobiol 19: 291–299.

Ince PG, Shaw PJ, Candy JM et al. (1994) Iron, selenium and glutathione peroxidase activity are elevated in sporadic motor neuron disease. Neurosci Lett 183: 87–90.

Ince PG, Shaw PJ, Slade JY, Jones C, Hudgson P (1996) Familial amyotrophic lateral sclerosis with a mutation in exon 4 of the Cu/Zn superoxide dismutase gene: pathological and immunocytochemical changes. Acta Neuropath 92: 395–403.

Ince PG, Shaw PJ, Lowe J (1998a) Motor neuron disease: recent advances in molecular pathology, pathogenesis and classification. Neuropathol Appl Neurobiol 24: 104–117.

Ince PG, Tomkins J, Slade JY, Thatcher NM, Shaw PJ (1998b) Amyotrophic lateral sclerosis associated with genetic abnormalities in the gene encoding Cu/Zn superoxide dismutase: molecular pathology of five new cases, and comparison with previous reports and 73 sporadic cases of ALS. J Neuropathol Exp Neurol 57: 895–904.

Iwanaga K, Hayashi S, Oyake M et al. (1997) Neuropathology of sporadic amyotrophic lateral sclerosis of long duration. J Neurol Sci 146: 139–143.

Kew JJM, Goldstein LH, Leigh PN et al. (1993a) The relationship between abnormalities of cognitive function and cerebral activation in amyotrophic lateral sclerosis. Brain 116: 1399–1423.

Kew JJM, Leigh PN, Playford ED et al. (1993b) Cortical function in amyotrophic lateral sclerosis: A positron emission tomography study. Brain 116: 644–680.

Klivenyi P, Ferrante RJ, Matthews RT et al. (1999) Neuroprotective effects of creatine in a transgenic animal model of amyotrophic lateral sclerosis. Nature Med 5: 347–350.

Kong J, Xu Z (1998) Massive mitochondrial degeneration in motor neurons triggers the onset of amyotrophic lateral sclerosis in mice expressing a mutant SOD1. J Neurosci 18: 3241–3250.

Kostic V, Jackson-Lewis V, de Bilbao F, Dubois-Dauphin M, Przedborski S (1997) Bcl-2: prolonging life in a transgenic mouse model of familial amyotrophic lateral sclerosis. Science 277: 559–562.

Krieger C, Lanius RA, Pelech SL, Shaw CA (1996) Amyotrophic lateral sclerosis: the involvement of intracellular calcium and protein kinase C. Trends Pharmacol Sci 17: 114–120.

Laake JH, Slyngstad TA, Haug F-MS, Ottersen OP (1995) Glutamine from glial cells is essential for the maintenance of the nerve terminal pool of glutamate: immunogold evidence from hippocampal slice cultures. J Neurochem 65: 871–881.

Lacomblez L, Bensimon G, Leigh PN et al. (1996) Dose-ranging study of riluzole in amyotrophic lateral sclerosis. Lancet 347: 1425–1432.

Lafon-Cazal M, Pietri S, Culcasi M et al. (1993) NMDA-dependent superoxide production and neurotoxicity. Nature 364: 535–537.

Lee MK, Marszalek JR, Cleveland DW (1994) A mutant neurofilament subunit causes massive, selective motor neuron death: implications for the pathogenesis of human motor neuron disease. Neuron 13: 975–988.

Lees GJ (1993) Contributory mechanisms in the causation of neurodegenerative disorders. Neuroscience 54: 287–322.

Leigh PN, Meldrum BS (1996) Excitotoxicity in ALS. Neurology 47 (Suppl 4): S221–S227.

Leigh PN, Dodson A, Swash M, Brion J-P, Anderton BH (1989) Cytoskeletal abnormalities in motor neuron disease: an immunocytochemical study. Brain 112: 521–535.

Li JH, Grynspan F, Berman S, Nixon R, Bursztajn S (1996) Regional differences in gene expression for calcium activated neutral proteases (calpains) and their endogenous inhibitor calpastatin in mouse brain and spinal cord. J Neurobiol 30: 177–191.

Lin CLG, Bristol LA, Dykes-Hoberg M, Crawford T, Clawson L, Rothstein JD (1998) Aberrant RNA processing in a neurodegenerative disease: the cause for absent EAAT2, a glutamate transporter in amyotrophic lateral sclerosis. Neuron 20: 589–602.

Linnane AW, Marzuki S, Ozawa T, Tanaka M (1989) Mitochondrial DNA mutations as an important contribution to ageing and degenerative diseases. Lancet 642–645.

Lupas A (1996) Coiled coils: new structures and new functions. Trends Biol Sci 21: 375–382.

Maher P, Davis JB (1996) The role of monoamine metabolism in oxidative glutamate toxicity. J Neurosci 16: 6394–6401.

Malessa S, Leigh PN, Bertel O, Sluga E, Hornykiewicz O (1991) Amyotrophic lateral sclerosis: glutamate dehydrogenase and transmitter amino acids in the spinal cord. J Neurol Neurosurg Psychiatr 54: 984–988.

Malgouris C, Daniel M, Doble A (1994) Neuroprotective effects of riluzole on N-methyl-D-aspartate-or veratridine-induced neurotoxicity in rat hippocampal slices. Neurosci Lett 177: 95–99.

Manetto V, Sternberger NH, Perry G, Sternberger LA, Gambetti P (1988) Phosphorylation of neurofilaments is altered in amyotrophic lateral sclerosis. J Neuropathol Exp Neurol 47: 642–653.

Matthews RT, Yang L, Browne S, Baik M, Beal MF (1998) Coenzyme Q_{10} administration increases brain mitochondrial concentrations and exerts neuroprotective effects. Proc Natl Acad Sci 95: 8892–8897.

Mattson MP, Guthrie PB, Kater SB (1989) A role for Na^+-dependent Ca^{++} extrusion in protection against neuronal excitotoxicity. FASEB J 3: 2519–2526.

Meccoci P, MacGarvey U, Kaufman AE et al. (1993) Oxidative damage to mitochondrial DNA shows marked age-dependent increases in human brain. Ann Neurol 34: 609–616.

Meldrum B, Garthwaite J (1990) Excitatory amino acid neurotoxicity and neurodegenerative disease. Trends Pharmacol Sci 11: 379–387.

Mena MA, Khan U, Togasaki DM, Sulzer D, Epstein CJ, Przedborski S (1997) Effects of wild-type and mutated copper/zinc superoxide dismutase on neuronal survival and L-DOPA induced toxicity in postnatal midbrain culture. J Neurochem 69: 21–33.

Miller RJ, Murphy SN, Glaum SR (1989) Neuronal Ca^{2+} channels and their regulation by excitatory amino acids. Ann NY Acad Sci 568: 149–158.

Mills KR (1995) Motor neuron disease: studies of the corticospinal excitation of single motoneurons by magnetic brain stimulation. Brain 118: 971–902.

Milton ID, Banner SJ, Ince PG et al. (1997) The immunohistochemical expression of the glial glutamate transporter EAAT2 in the human CNS. Mol Brain Res 52: 17–31.

Molander C, Xu Q, Rivero-Mellian C, Grant G (1989) Cytoarchitectonic organisation of the spinal cord in the rat. II The cervical and thoracic cord. J Comp Neurol 289: 375–385.

Munoz DG, Green C, Perl D, Selkoe DJ (1988) Accumulation of phosphorylated neurofilaments in anterior horn motoneurons of ALS patients. J Neuropathol Exp Neurol 47: 9–18.

Murayama S, Ookawa Y, Mori H et al. (1989) Immunocytochemical and ultrastructural study of Lewy-body-like inclusions in familial amyotrophic lateral sclerosis. Acta Neuropath 78: 143–152.

Murphy TH, Miyamoto M, Sastre A, Schnaar RL, Coyle JT (1989) Glutamate toxicity in a neuronal cell line involves inhibition of cystine transport leading to oxidative stress. Neuron 22: 1547–1558.

Nagai M, Abe K, Okamoto K, Itoyama Y (1998) Identification of alternative splicing forms of GLT-1 mRNA in the spinal cord of amyotrophic lateral sclerosis patients. Neurosci Lett 244: 165–168.

Nixon RA, Shea TB (1992) Dynamics of neuronal intermediate filaments: a developmental perspective. Cell Motil Cytoskeleton 22: 81–91.

Novelli A, Reilly JA, Lysko PG, Henneberry RC (1988) Glutamate becomes neurotoxic via the N-methyl-D-aspartate receptor when intracellular energy levels are reduced. Brain Res 451: 205–212.

O'Brien RJ, Fischbach GD (1986) Characterisation of excitatory amino acid receptors expressed by chick motor neurons in vitro. J Neurosci 6: 3290–3296.

Olanow CW (1993) A radical hypothesis for neurodegeneration. Trends Neurol Sci 16: 439–444.

Olkowski ZL (1998) Mutant AP endonuclease in patients with amyotrophic lateral sclerosis. NeuroReport 9: 239–242.

Olney JW (1978) Neurotoxicity of excitatory amino acids. In: McGeer EG, Olney JW, McGeer P (eds). Kainic Acid as a Tool in Neurobiology. Raven Press: New York, pp. 95–121.

Orrenius S, McConkey DJ, Bellomo G, Nicotera P (1989) Role of Ca^{++} in toxic cell killing. Trends Pharmacol Sci 10: 281–284.

Pardo CA, Xu Z, Borchelt DR, Price DL, Sisodia SS, Cleveland DW (1995) Superoxide dismutase is an abundant component in cell bodies, dendrites and axons of motor neurons and in a subset of other neurons. Proc Natl Acad Sci 92(4): 954–958.

Pelligrini-Giampietro DE (1994) Free radicals and the pathogenesis of neuronal death: cooperative role of excitatory amino acids. In: Armstrong D (ed.) Free Radicals in Diagnostic Medicine. Plenum: New York, pp. 59–71.

Perry TL, Hansen S, Jones K (1987) Brain glutamate deficiency in amyotrophic lateral sclerosis. Neurology 37: 1845–1848.

Perry TL, Krieger C, Hansen S, Eisen A (1990) Amyotrophic lateral sclerosis: amino acid levels in plasma and cerebrospinal fluid. Ann Neurol 28: 12–17.

Phillips JP, Tainer JA, Getzoff ED et al. (1995) Subunit-destabilising mutations in Drosophila copper/zinc superoxide dismutase: neuropathology and a model of dimer dysequilibrium. Proc Natl Acad Sci USA 92: 8533–8534.

Plaitakis A, Caroscio JT (1987) Abnormal glutamate metabolism in amyotrophic lateral sclerosis. Ann Neurol 22: 575–579.

Plaitakis A, Constantakakis E, Smith J (1988) The neuroexcitotoxic amino acids glutamate and aspartate are altered in the spinal cord and brain in amyotrophic lateral sclerosis. Ann Neurol 24: 446–449.

Przedborski S, Donaldson D, Jakowec M et al. (1996) Brain superoxide dismutase, catalase and glutathione peroxidase activities in amyotrophic lateral sclerosis. Ann Neurol 39: 158–165.

Rabizadeh S, Ralla EB, Borchelt DR et al. (1995) Mutations associated with amyotrophic lateral sclerosis convert superoxide dismutase from an antiapoptotic gene to a proapoptotic gene: studies in yeast and neural cells. Proc Natl Acad Sci 92: 3024–3028.

Radunovic A, Leigh PN (1996) Cu/Zn superoxide dismutase gene mutations in amyotrophic lateral sclerosis: correlation between genotype and clinical features. J Neurol Neurosurg Psychiatry 61: 565–572.

Reaume AG, Elliot JL, Hoffman EK et al. (1996) Motor neurons in Cu/Zn superoxide dismutase-deficient mice develop normally but exhibit enhanced cell death after axonal injury. Nature Genet 13: 43–47.

Richter C (1995) Oxidative damage to mitochondrial DNA and its relationship to ageing. Int J Biochem Cell Biol 27: 647–653.

Richter C, Park JW, Ames BN (1988) Normal oxidative damage to mitochondrial and nuclear DNA is extensive. Proc Natl Acad Sci USA 85: 6465–6467.

Ripps ME, Huntley GW, Hof PR, Morrison JH, Gordon JW (1995) Transgenic mice expressing an altered murine superoxide dismutase gene provide an animal model of amyotrophic lateral sclerosis. Proc Natl Acad Sci 92(3): 689–693.

Rosen DR, Siddique T, Patterson D et al. (1993) Mutations in Cu/Zn superoxide dismutase are associated with familial amyotrophic lateral sclerosis. Nature 362: 59–62.

Rothstein JD (1995) Excitotoxic mechanisms in the pathogenesis of amyotrophic lateral sclerosis. Adv Neurol 68: 7–20.

Rothstein JD (1996) Excitotoxicity and neurodegeneration in amyotropic lateral sclerosis. Clin Neurosci 3: 348–359.

Rothstein JD, Kuncl RW (1995) Neuroprotective strategies in a model of chronic glutamate-mediated motor neuron toxicity. J Neurochem 65: 643–651.

Rothstein JD, Tsai G, Kuncl RW et al. (1990) Abnormal excitatory amino acid metabolism in amyotrophic lateral sclerosis. Ann Neurol 28: 18–25.

Rothstein JD, Kuncl RW, Chaudhry V et al. (1991) Excitatory amino acids in amyotrophic lateral sclerosis: an update. Ann Neurol 30: 224–225.

Rothstein JD, Martin LJ, Kuncl RW (1992) Decreased glutamate transport by the brain and spinal cord in amyotrophic lateral sclerosis. New Engl J Med 326: 1464–1468.

Rothstein JD, Jin L, Dykes-Hoberg M, Kuncl RW (1993) Chronic inhibition of glutamate uptake produces a model of slow neurotoxicity. Proc Natl Acad Sci 90: 6591–6595.

Rothstein JD, Bristol LA, Hosler B, Brown RH, Kuncl RW (1994a) Chronic inhibition of superoxide dismutase produces apoptotic death of spinal neurons. Proc Natl Acad Sci USA 91: 4155–4159.

Rothstein JD, Martin L, Levey AI et al. (1994b) Localization of neuronal and glial glutamate transporters. Neuron 13: 713–725.

Rothstein JD, Van Kammen M, Levey AI, Martin LJ, Kuncl RW (1995) Selective loss of glial glutamate transporter GLT-1 in amyotrophic lateral sclerosis. Ann Neurol 38: 73–84.

Rothstein JD, Dykes-Hoberg M, Pardo CA et al. (1996) Knockout of glutamate transporters reveals a major role for astroglial transport in excitotoxicity and clearance of glutamate. Neuron 16: 675–686.

Rouleau GA, Clark AW, Rooke K et al. (1996) SOD1 mutation is associated with accumulation of neurofilaments in amyotrophic lateral sclerosis. Ann Neurol 39: 128–131.

Schor NF (1988) Inactivation of mammalian brain glutamine synthetase by oxygen radicals. Brain Res 456: 17–21.

Schousboe A, Westergaard N, Sonnewald U (1993) Glutamate and glutamine metabolism and compartmentation in astrocytes. Dev Neurosci 15: 359–366.

Shaw CE, Enayat ZE, Chioza BA et al. (1998a) Mutations in all five exons of SOD-1 may cause ALS. Ann Neurol 43: 390–394.

Shaw PJ (1994) Excitotoxicity and motor neuron disease: a review of the evidence. J Neurol Sci 124(suppl): 6–13.

Shaw PJ (1998) Excitotoxicity, genetics and neurodegeneration in amyotrophic lateral sclerosis. In: Seeburg PH, Bresink I, Turski L (eds). Ernst Schering Research Foundation Workshop 23. Excitatory Amino Acids: from Genes to Therapy. Springer: Berlin; pp. 65–94.

Shaw PJ, Ince PG (1994) A quantitative autoradiographic study of [³H]kainate binding sites in the normal spinal cord, brainstem and motor cortex. Brain Res 641: 39–45.

Shaw PJ, Ince PG (1997) Glutamate, excitotoxicity and amyotrophic lateral sclerosis. J Neurol 244 (Suppl 2): S3–S14.

Shaw PJ, Ince PG, Johnson M, Perry EK, Candy JM (1991) The quantitative autoradiographic distribution of [³H]MK-801 binding sites in the normal human spinal cord. Brain Res 539: 164–168.

Shaw PJ, Chinnery RM, Ince PG (1994a) Non-NMDA receptors in motor neuron disease (MND): a quantitative study in spinal cord and motor cortex using [³H]CNQX and [³H]kainate. Brain Res 655: 186–194.

Shaw PJ, Chinnery RM, Ince PG (1994b) [³H]D-Aspartate binding sites in the normal human spinal cord and changes in motor neuron disease: a quantitative autoradiographic study. Brain Res 655: 195–201.

Shaw PJ, Ince PG, Matthews JNS, Johnson M, Candy JM (1994c) N-Methyl-D-aspartate (NMDA) receptors in the spinal cord and motor cortex in motor neuron disease: a quantitative autoradiographic study using [³H]MK-801. Brain Res 637: 297–302.

Shaw PJ, Forrest V, Ince PG, Richardson JP, Wastell HJ (1995a) CSF and plasma amino acid levels in motor neuron disease: elevation of CSF glutamate in a subset of patients. Neurodegeneration 4: 209–216.

Shaw PJ, Ince PG, Falkous G, Mantle D (1995b) Oxidative damage to protein in sporadic motor neuron disease spinal cord. Ann Neurol 38: 691–695.

Shaw PJ, Chinnery RM, Thagesen H, Borthwick G, Ince PG (1997a) Immunocytochemical study of the distribution of the free radical scavenging enzymes Cu/Zn superoxide dismutase (SOD1), Mn superoxide dismutase (Mn SOD) and catalase in the normal human spinal cord and in motor neuron disease. J Neurol Sci 147: 115–125.

Shaw PJ, Tomkins J, Slade JY et al. (1997b) CNS tissue Cu/Zn superoxide dismutase (SOD1) mutations in motor neuron disease (MND). NeuroReport 8: 3923–3927.

Shaw PJ, Williams TL, Slade JY, Eggett CJ, Ince PG (1999) Low expression of GluR2 AMPA receptor subunit protein by human motor neurons. NeuroReport 10: 261–265.

Shibata N, Hirano A, Kobayashi A et al. (1993) Immunohistochemical demonstration of Cu/Zn superoxide dismutase in the spinal cord of patients with familial amyotrophic lateral sclerosis. Acta Histochem Cytochem 26: 619–622.

Siddique T, Nijhawan D, Hentat A (1996) Molecular genetic basis of familial ALS. Neurol 47 (suppl 2): S27–S35.

Siesjo BK (1988) Historical overview. Calcium, ischaemia and death of brain cells. Ann NY Acad Sci 522: 638–661.

Siesjo BK (1994) Calcium-mediated processes in neuronal degeneration. Ann NY Acad Sci 747: 140–161.

Siklos L, Engelhardt J, Harati Y, R.G. S, Joo F, Appel SH (1996) Ultrastructural evidence for altered calcium in motor nerve terminals in amyotrophic lateral sclerosis. Ann Neurol 39: 203–219.

Siklos L, Engelhardt JI, Alexianu ME, Gurney ME, Siddique T, Appel SH (1998) Intracellular calcium parallels motoneuron degeneration in SOD-1 mutant mice. J Neuropath Exp Neurol 57: 571–587.

Sillevis Smitt PAE, Mulder TPJ, Verspaget HW, Blaauwgeers HGT, Troost D, de Jong JMBV (1994) Metallothionein in amyotrophic lateral sclerosis. Biol Signals 3(4): 193–197.

Smith RG, Appel SH (1995) Molecular approaches to amyotrophic lateral sclerosis. Annu Rev Med 46: 133–145.

Smith RG, Henry YK, Mattson MP, Appel SH (1998) Presence of 4-hydroxynonenal in cerebrospinal fluid of patients with sporadic amyotrophic lateral sclerosis. Ann Neurol 44: 696–699.

Sobue G, Hashizume Y, Yasuda T (1990) Phosphorylated high molecular weight neurofilament protein in lower motor neurons in ALS and other neurodegenerative diseases involving ventral horn cells. Acta Neuropathol 79: 402–408.

Sommer B, Seeburg PH (1992) Glutamate receptor channels: novel properties and new clones. Trends Pharmacol Sci 13: 291–296.

Subramaniam JJ, Yiannikas C (1990) Multimodality evoked potentials in motor neuron disease. Arch Neurol 47: 989–994.

Susel Z, Engber TM, Kuo S, Chase TN (1991) Prolonged infusion of quinolinic acid into rat striatum as an excitotoxic model of neurodegenerative disease. Neurosci Lett 121: 234–238.

Tomkins J, Usher PA, Slade JY et al. (1998) Novel insertion in the KSP repeat region of the heavy neurofilament gene in amyotrophic lateral sclerosis. NeuroReport 9: 3967–3970.

Traynelis SF, Hartley M, Heinemann SF (1995) Control of proton sensitivity of the NMDA receptor by RNA splicing and polyamines. Science 268: 873–876.

Troy CM, Shelanski M (1994) Down regulation of copper/zinc superoxide dismutase causes apoptotic death in PC12 neuronal cells. Proc Natl Acad Sci USA 91: 6384–6387.

Trotti D, Aoki M, Pasinelli P, et al. (2001) Amyotrophic lateral sclerosis-linked glutamate transporter mutant has impaired glutamate clearance capacity. J Biol Chem 276: 576–582.

Tsai G, Stauch-Slusher B, Sim L et al. (1991) Reductions in acidic amino acids and N-acetyl-aspartyl glutamate (NAAG) in amyotrophic lateral sclerosis CNS. Brain Res 655: 195–201.

Tu PH, Raju P, Robinson KA, Gurney ME, Trojanowski JQ, Lee VM (1996) Transgenic mice carrying a human mutant superoxide dismutase transgene develop neuronal cytoskeletal pathology resembling human amyotrophic lateral sclerosis lesions. Proc Natl Acad Sci USA 93: 3155–3160.

Volterra A, Trott D, Cassutti P et al. (1992) High sensitivity of glutamate uptake to extracellular free arachidonic acid levels in rat cortical synaptosomes and astrocytes. J Neurochem 59: 600–606.

Volterra A, Trott D, Racagni G (1994) Glutamate uptake is inhibited by arachidonic acid and oxygen radicals via two distinct and additive mechanisms. Mol Pharmacol 46: 986–992.

Wang X, Culotta VC, Klee CB (1996) Superoxide dismutase protects calcineurin from inactivation. Nature 383: 434–437.

Westbrook GL (1994) Glutamate receptor update. Curr Opin Neurobiol 4: 337–346.

Wiedau-Pazos M, Goto JJ, Rabizadeh S et al. (1996) Altered reactivity of superoxide dismutase in familial amyotrophic lateral sclerosis. Science 271: 515–518.

Williams TL, Shaw PJ, Lowe J, Bates D, Ince PG (1995) Parkinsonism in motor neuron disease: case report and literature review. Acta Neuropathol 89: 275–283.

Williams TL, Ince PG, Oakley AE, Shaw PJ (1996) An immunocytochemical study of the distribution of AMPA selective glutamate receptor subunits in the normal human motor system. Neuroscience 74: 185–198.

Williams TL, Day NC, Ince PG, Kamboj RK, Shaw PJ (1997) Calcium-permeable alpha-amino-3-hydroxy-5-methyl-4-isoxazole propionic acid receptors: a molecular determinant of selective vulnerability in amyotrophic lateral sclerosis. Ann Neurol 42: 200–207.

Wong PC, Pardo CA, Borchelt DR et al. (1995) An adverse property of a familial ALS-linked SOD1 mutation causes motor neuron disease characterized by vacuolar degeneration of mitochondria. Neuron 14(6): 1105–1116.

Xu Z, Cork L, Griffin J, Cleveland D (1993) Increased expression of neurofilament subunit NF-L produces morphological alterations that resemble the pathology of human motor neuron disease. Cell 73: 23–33.

Yim HS, Kang JH, Chock PB, Stadtman ER, Yim MB (1997) A familial amyotrophic lateral sclerosis associated A4V Cu/Zn superoxide dismutase mutant has a lower Km for hydrogen peroxide. J Biol Chem 272: 8861–8863.

Young AB, Penney JB (1992) Pharmacological aspects of motor dysfunction. In: Asbury AK, McKham GM, McDonald WI (eds). Diseases of the Nervous System, Clinical Neurobiology. Volume 1. WB Saunders: Philadelphia, pp. 342–352.

Young AB, Penney JB, Dauth GW, Bramberg MB, Gilman S (1983) Glutamate or aspartate as a possible neurotransmitter of cerebral corticofugal fibres in the monkey. Neurol 33: 1513–1516.

Zeman S, Lloyd C, Meldrum B, Leigh PN (1994) Excitatory amino acids, free radicals and the pathogenesis of motor neuron disease. Neuropathol Appl Neurobiol 20: 219–231.

Zhang Y, Marcillat O, Giulivi C, Ernster L, Davies KJA (1990) The oxidative inactivation of mitochondrial electron transport chain components and ATPase. J Biol Chem 265: 16330–16336.

Zhang B, Tu P, Abtahian F, Trojanowski JQ, Lee VMY (1997) Neurofilaments and orthograde transport are reduced in ventral roots of transgenic mice that express human SOD1 with a G93A mutation. J Cell Biol 5: 1307–1315.

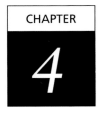

Genetics of familial amyotrophic lateral sclerosis and ethical aspects

Wim Robberecht, MD, PhD

Most patients with amyotrophic lateral sclerosis (ALS) are considered to have sporadic ALS (SALS). In a minority of cases, the condition is familial (FALS) and then most commonly inherited as an autosomal dominant trait. Autosomal recessive FALS is rare. An X-linked form has been delineated recently.

Autosomal dominant FALS (AD-FALS)

ALS is transmitted as an autosomal dominant disease in about 5 to 10% of ALS patients (Mulder et al., 1986; Haverkamp et al., 1995). Autosomal dominant FALS (AD-FALS) is clinically and pathologically very similar to SALS (Mulder et al., 1986; Li et al., 1988; Veltema et al., 1990). Site of onset can be limb, trunk or bulbar, but the latter appears to be less frequent in FALS than SALS (Cudkowicz et al., 1997; Radunovic and Leigh, 1996). The degree of upper motor neuron involvement is as variable as it is in SALS, and within a family, patients with both lower and upper motor neuron signs, only lower motor neuron signs, and (almost) only upper motor neuron signs can be found. Onset appears to be somewhat earlier in AD-FALS than in SALS (Mulder et al., 1986; Haverkamp et al., 1995), but variation is as large as in SALS. Penetrance is age-dependent. Fifty percent of patients are affected at the age of 46 and 90% at the age of 70 (Strong et al., 1991). Some authors suggest extra-motor neuron involvement (such as abnormalities of the posterior column, spinocerebellar tract and Clarke's column) to be more frequent in FALS, both clinically and pathologically (Hirano et al., 1967; Metcalf & Hirano et al., 1971; Bobowick & Brody et al., 1973; Li et al., 1988; Veltema et al., 1990; Andersen et al., 1996; Kawata et al., 1997).

SOD1-associated AD-FALS (*SOD1*-FALS)

In 1991, linkage between FALS and chromosome 21q22.1-22.2 was reported (Siddique et al., 1991). Subsequently, mutations in the *SOD1* gene were identified, which represented a major breakthrough for ALS research (Rosen et al., 1993). It is now known that such mutations underly the disease in about 20% of families (Cudkowicz et al., 1997; Orrell et al., 1997; Shaw et al., 1998). *SOD1* encodes the copper- and zinc-dependent superoxide dismutase SOD1. This cytosolic enzyme converts superoxide anions ($O_2^{\bullet-}$) into hydrogen peroxide (H_2O_2) (Figure 4.1) (Fridovich, 1986). This H_2O_2 is then further metabolized into H_2O and O_2 by glutathione peroxidase. SOD1 thus plays an essential role in free radical scavenging.

Biology of *SOD1*-FALS

The *SOD1* gene spans about 11 kb of genomic DNA on chromosome 21 (Levanon et al., 1985). It consists of 5 exons, separated by 4 introns, and is highly conserved. It is expressed constitutively and ubiquitously. It generates 2 mRNA species (0.7 and 0.9 kb).

The SOD1 monomere consists of 153 aminoacids, which are organized in 8 antiparallel β-strands arranged in two interlocking Greek key motifs forming a β-barrel (Getzoff et al., 1989). The apoenzyme binds one Cu^{2+} and one

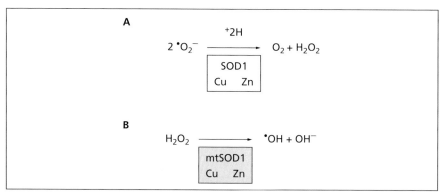

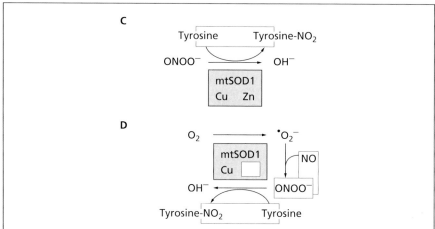

Fig. 4.1 Schematic representation of the normal function of SOD1 (white box) (panel A) and the hypothetical mechanism explaining the gain of function of the mutated SOD1 (grey box): peroxidase activity (panel B), nitration of tyrosine residues (panel C), and nitration of tyrosines after generation of superoxide anions through reversal of the catalytic process due to loss of Zn from the enzyme (panel D.)

Zn^{2+} ion, and functions as a homodimer, although the two active sites seem to operate independently. The aminoacid residues critical for the conformation of the protein and for the non-covalent dimer interaction are well identified. Two stretches of aminoacids form an electrostatically active tunnel leading to the Cu^{2+} ion in the active center of the enzyme (residues G44-D83 and H120-C146) (Getzoff et al., 1989; Deng et al., 1993). This channel is 24 Å in diameter at the surface but gradually narrows to 10 Å. Substrate specificity is determined by the electrostatic and steric interactions in this tunnel. Residue H63 and the Cu^{2+} ion are essential for the dismutase reaction, while Zn^{2+} appears to be essential for the dissociation of the H_2O_2 formed and the pH stability of the reaction.

Over 90 mutations have been reported to be associated with ALS at the time of writing; they have been recently reviewed (Andersen, 2000). An up-to-date overview of all mutations reported and their references can be found at *www.alsod.org*. Mutations have been found in all five exons, although only few have been identified in exon 3, which encodes the active center of the enzyme. In the US, the most frequent mutation is the A4V mutation, being present in about 50% of families (Rosen et al., 1994; Juneja et al., 1997; Cudkowicz et al., 1997). All but one (see below) of the mutations described behave as dominant traits, making inactivation or absence of the enzyme an unlikely explanation for the motor neuron death these mutations induce. Furthermore, most of the mutations identified so far have been single base pair changes (point mutations), resulting in a substitution of aminoacids (missense mutations), giving rise to a rather subtle structural or conformational change (Deng et al., 1993). A few short insertions or deletions have been reported to occur at the end of intron 4 or the beginning of exon 5, resulting in the expression of a protein missing the terminal stretch of aminoacids (*www.alsod.org*). Mutations resulting in the complete absence of the protein have not been reported so far. This suggests that the bigger part of the protein needs to be present to give rise to the process leading to ALS.

Most of the mutations result in a variable loss of dismutase activity of the mutated SOD1 (Deng et al., 1993; Bowling et al., 1993; Robberecht et al., 1994; Bowling et al., 1995). However, some (e.g. the D90A and the G37R mutation) do not affect the enzymatic activity at all and still give rise to ALS (Bowling et al., 1995; Andersen et al., 1995; Själander et al., 1995). There is no correlation between the phenotype and the residual dismutase activity (Bowling et al., 1995). Furthermore, transgenic mice overexpressing a human mutated *SOD1* gene develop an ALS-like motor neuron disease, despite normal or elevated cellular dismutase activity (Gurney et al., 1994; Ripps, 1995; Wong, 1995; Bruijn et al., 1997). Mice in which the *SOD1* gene has been knocked out, on the other hand, do not develop spontaneous motor neuron loss (Reaume, 1996). Because of all these arguments, it is the current thinking that the mutated SOD1 acquires a new cytotoxic activity (*gain of function*).

This newly acquired activity remains unidentified so far. Several hypotheses have been formulated (Figure 4.2) (Brown Jr and Robberecht, 2001; Cleveland Rothstein, 2001). An abnormal tendency to form aggregates, and an aberrant biochemical activity are the most investigated ones. The latter hypothesis suggests that the mutations induce a structural change in the protein's conformation, so

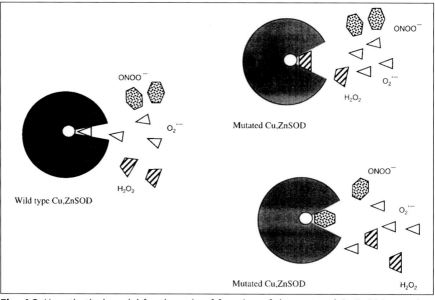

Fig. 4.2 Hypothetical model for the gain of function of the mutated Cu,ZnSOD protein: 'abnormal' substrates gain access to the active center due to slight conformational changes induced by the single amino acid mutations

that substrates other than $O_2^{\bullet-}$ gain access to its active center (Figure 4.2). Some (Wiedau-Pazos et al., 1996; Yim et al., 1997), but not all (Singh et al., 1998) biochemical studies have demonstrated that the mutated enzyme's affinity for H_2O_2 is increased. It could thus function as a peroxidase and use H_2O_2 as a substrate to generate toxic hydroxyl radicals ($OH^{\bullet}$). Enhanced $OH^{\bullet}$ production (Bogdanov et al., 1998) or increased free radical production in general (Liu et al., 1998) has indeed been demonstrated in mutant *SOD1* mouse brain. Other researchers have suggested that the mutated SOD1 induces the nitration of tyrosine residues by generating nitronium ions (NO_2^+) from peroxynitrate ($ONOO^-$) (Beckman et al., 1993). This $ONOO^-$ comes from the reaction of $O_2^{\bullet-}$ with NO, generated from L-arginine by NO synthase. According to a related hypothesis, the mutated enzyme's affinity for Zn^{2+} is reduced (Crow et al., 1997; Estevez et al., 1999). The Zn^{2+}-depleted enzyme allows rapid reduction of the Cu^{2+} to Cu^+, resulting in reversal of the catalytic cycle giving rise to the formation of $O_2^{\bullet-}$ from O_2. This $O_2^{\bullet-}$ could then react with NO to form $ONOO^-$, again inducing nitration of tyrosines.

Although these hypotheses remain unproven, evidence for nitration of tyrosines (Abe et al., 1995; Bruijn et al., 1997; Beal et al., 1997; Ferrante et al., 1997), for free radical-induced damage of proteins, lipids and nucleic acids (Bowling et al., 1993; Shaw et al., 1995; Andrus et al., 1998; Pedersen et al., 1998; Hall et al., 1998), and for increased sensitivity to oxidative stress (Aguirre et al., 1998) has been found in tissue of both mice and humans with mutant SOD1-induced motor neuron degeneration. Indirect evidence for the role of oxidative stress is also provided by the finding that treatment of the *SOD1* transgenic mice with antioxidants delays onset of clinical disease (Gurney et al., 1996)).

For all these reasons, it seems likely that oxidative damage somehow plays a pathogenic role (for review see Robberecht, 2000). Of major interest is the finding that oxidative stress and excitotoxicity may be linked through mutant SOD1-induced damage of EAAT2, the main astrocytic glutamate transporter (Trotti et al., 1999) (see below and elsewhere in this issue).

According to the alternative hypothesis, the mutated SOD1 tends to form intracellular aggregates (Bruijn et al., 1997; Bruijn et al., 1998). This aggregation is supposed to occur when the ubiquitin- and proteasome-dependent degradation of the mutated protein is being overwhelmed by the amount of mutated SOD1 protein. The cytotoxic effect of this aggregation may result from either coaggregation of necessary cellular constituents, inhibition of normal proteasomic function, or a mechanical or biochemical action of the aggregates themselves (Cleveland and Rothstein, 2001). A possible example of such action may be an inhibition of axonal transport, called axonal strangulation (Borchelt et al., 1998; Williamson and Cleveland, 1999). The concept that misfolding of SOD1 is involved in the pathogenesis of ALS is supported by the *in vitro* finding that heat shock proteins may protect motor neurons from mutant SOD1-induced cell death (Bruening et al., 1999).

SOD1-FALS phenotype

SOD1-FALS does not appear to have any substantial clinical characteristics distinguishing it from non-*SOD1*-FALS or indeed SALS (Juneja et al., 1997; Cudkowicz et al., 1997). Onset of *SOD1*-FALS averages between 45 and 50 years of age, but varies between 15 and 81 years. In the patients reported, the onset of FALS associated with the G37R and L38V mutations is earlier (mean age of onset was 29.3 ± 1.2 years for G37R). Penetrance is age-dependent. In a large study by Cudkowicz et al., 92% of patients were affected by the age of 70 (Cudkowicz et al., 1997). We found a similar result in our mutated *SOD1*-associated FALS patients: as shown in Figure 4.3, 50% of patients were affected by the age of 43, while 97% were affected by the age of 70 years (Vanopdenbosch and Robberecht, 2001). It looks as if penetrance of *SOD1* mutations is high. For the A4V mutation it is estimated to be 91%, and 100% for the L38V, E100G

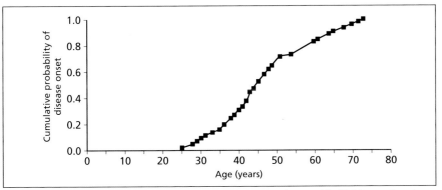

Fig. 4.3 Cumulative probability of disease onset in 34 patients with *SOD1*-associated FALS.

and I113T (Cudkowicz et al., 1997). However, others have suggested incomplete penetrance for A4T and I113T (Suthers et al., 1994; Nakano et al., 1994; Radunovic & Leigh, 1996). *SOD1*-FALS is clinically characterized by lower motor neuron signs with a variable degree of upper motor neuron signs. Patients with the A4V mutation have lower motor neuron signs only (Rosen et al., 1994; Andersen et al., 1997; Cudkowicz et al., 1998). Even on pathological examination axonal loss in the corticospinal tract is usually mild or absent in patients with this mutation. The G93C mutation is mainly characterized by lower motor neuron signs as well (Vanopdenbosch and Robberecht, 2001).

There is quite some variation in prognosis among the different mutations. The survival of *SOD1*-FALS patients in general is similar to that in SALS (Juneja et al., 1997; Cudkowicz et al., 1997). The A4V mutation is well known to induce a severe phenotype, with a survival of 1.4 years (Rosen et al., 1994; Juneja et al., 1997; Cudkowicz et al., 1997). By contrast, other mutations (e.g. E21G, G37R, G41D, H46R, D90A, G93C, G83V, I104F, L144S, I151T) are associated with surprisingly long survival of 10 years or even longer (Aoki et al., 1993; Aoki et al., 1994; Cudkowicz et al., 1997; Juneja et al., 1997; Vanopdenbosch & Robberecht, 2001).

This *interfamilial* variability, at least in part, may be due to differences in the effects of the different mutations on the newly acquired cytotoxic function of the mutated enzyme. Similarily important, however, is the *intrafamilial* phenotypic variation. The latter is quite obvious for the D90A mutation: for some patients the disease is fatal within one or two years, whereas other affected family members survive for more than 10 years (Robberecht et al., 1996). The same large variation is observed in families with the I113T mutation (Orrell et al., 1995). It is tempting to speculate on the existence of (a) factor(s), either environmental or genetic in nature, that modify(ies) phenotypic expression (see autosomal recessive FALS). The identification of these factors may be of major importance for possible preventive strategies.

AD-FALS not associated with *SOD1* mutations

It should be emphasized that in 4 out of 5 families with ALS, the disease is not associated with exonic mutations in *SOD1*. The genetic deficit underlying the motor neuron degeneration in these instances is unknown at the time of writing, but several loci are known to be linked to the disease (Table 4.1).

An autosomal dominant juvenile onset form with some particular features has been linked to chromosome 9q34 (Chance et al., 1998; Rabin et al., 1999). A form associated with frontal dementia has been linked to chromosome 9q21-22 (Hosler et al., 2000). A third locus associated with classical ALS has been identified on chromosome 18q (Hand et al., 2002). The identification of the underlying genes is awaited eagerly.

Autosomal recessive FALS (AR-FALS)

Hitherto, AR-FALS has been described in two instances: FALS associated with a D90A mutation in the *SOD1* gene in pedigrees of Scandinavian origin, and recessive juvenile onset FALS that has been reported in the Arabic population.

Table 4.1 Loci and genes associated with ALS

	Designation	Locus	Gene product	Mode of inheritance
Familial	ALS1	21q22.1-22.2	SOD1	dominant
	ALS2	2q33	alsin	recessive
	ALS3	18q	?	dominant
		?	?	dominant
	ALS4	9q34	?	dominant
	ALS5	15q15-22	?	recessive
	ALS Frontotemporal dementia	9q21-22	?	dominant
	—	17q21	tau	dominant
	—	Xp11-q12	?	dominant
Sporadic		22q12	NF-H	
		11p13	EAAT2	
		14q11	APEX nuclease	
		mitochondrial	Cytochrome c oxidase subunit I	
		?5q13 (*SMN2* deletions)	SMN	
		?5q13 (*SMN2* copy number)	SMN	

Autosomal recessive *SOD1*-FALS

FALS pedigrees of Scandinavian origin with autosomal recessive inheritance have been described extensively by Andersen et al., (Andersen et al., 1995; Andersen et al., 1996; Andersen et al., 1997). Most originated from the region of the river Torne in the north of Sweden and Finland. Surprisingly, the disease is associated with the D90A mutation in the *SOD1* gene. In these families only homozygous D90A individuals are affected by ALS. D90A heterozygosity is present in about 2.5% of individuals in that region, and is not associated with neurodegenerative disease.

The phenotype of D90A homozygous patients is stereotyped and unusual (Andersen et al., 1995; Andersen et al., 1996; Andersen et al., 1997). Upper and lower motor neurons appear to be involved, with the lower extremities affected predominantly. Age of onset varies between 20 and 94(!) years, and mean survival is 13 years, but can be more than 24 years(!). In several patients, clinical features such as mild ataxia, paresthesias, and micturition problems suggest extra-motor neuron involvement. Reflexes, hyperactive initially, disappear over time.

Similar D90A recessive pedigrees have been found in France and the US. However, as mentioned above, the D90A mutation has also been associated with AD-FALS (Robberecht et al., 1996), and ALS patients heterozygous for the D90A mutation have now been found in France, the UK and Australia. The D90A substitution can thus behave both as a recessive and dominant mutation. This is particularly intriguing as this mutation does not seem to affect the enzyme's activity (Andersen et al., 1995; Själander et al., 1995). It can be hypothesised that an unknown factor protects heterozygous individuals in the recessive pedigrees or, alternatively, that the susceptibility of heterozygous individuals in the dominant pedigrees is increased. Evidence for the existence of a genetic protective factor which modifies the deleterious effects of the mutant *SOD1* in the recessive families, has been suggested (Al-Chalabi et al., 1998). As mentioned above, the identification of such factor may be of importance to delineate a protective treatment strategy.

Recently, another SOD1 mutation, the D96N mutation, has been suggested to behave as a recessive trait as well (Hand, 2001). However, this report awaits confirmation, as dominant inheritance with reduced penetration remains to be excluded for this mutation.

Juvenile onset AR-FALS

Pedigrees with AR-FALS with onset in the first or second decade and with slow progression of symptoms have been extensively characterized by Hamida et al. (Hamida, 1990). Several clinical variants have been described: in some families weakness and atrophy (mainly in the upper extremities) is associated with upper motor neuron findings in all limbs (type 1), while in others, spasticity of the lower limbs is accompanied by amyotrophy of the peroneal muscles (type 2). Other families may be classified as having juvenile primary lateral sclerosis, as upper motor neuron signs predominate in the facial and limb muscles, with very mild or no lower motor neuron findings (type 3). Age of onset is around 12 years but varies from 3 to 23 years. The duration of the disease is 15 to 20 years. Consanguinity is found in several of the pedigrees described.

Two loci for autosomal recessive forms of juvenile ALS have been identified: one on chromosome 2q33-q35 (type 3) (Hentati et al., 1994) and the other one on chromosome 15q12-21 (type 1) (Hentati et al., 1998). The gene underlying motor neuron disease in the 2q33-35 locus has now been identified (Hadano et al., 2001; Yang et al., 2001). It encodes for alsin, a protein containing guanine-nucleotide exchange factor domains, the function of which needs further study. The gene product is alternatively spliced, resulting in a short and long form of alsin (Hadano et al., 2001; Yang et al., 2001). Mutations in the part of the gene encoding the sequence common to these two forms are associated with disease characterized by both upper and lower motor neuron signs (ALS), while mutations that are only expressed in the longer form of the protein give rise to a phenotype with upper motor neuron signs only (PLS) and with prolonged survival. How these mutations result in selective motor neuron death remains to be clarified. As this is a recessive disorder, loss of function of alsin is likely to be the underlying mechanism.

X-linked ALS

Surprisingly, a dominant form has been linked to chromosome Xp11-q12 (Siddique et al., 1998a). The underlying gene has not been identified.

Other familial ALS syndromes

Autosomal dominant frontotemporal dementia and parkinsonism associated with mutations in the tau gene on chromosome 17q21 is accompanied by amyotrophy (Lynch et al., 1994; Hutton et al., 1998; Spillantini et al., 1998). This suggests the importance of the tau protein to the biology and pathology of motor neurons. Support for this comes from the finding that mice overexpressing the four repeat-containing form of human tau or a mutated tau develop a motor axonopathy (Spittaels et al., 1999; Lewis et al., 2000). Hirayama's disease is a focal and non-progressive amyotrophy of the upper limb, occuring in young adults. Its pathogenesis is unknown, and rare familial cases have been described. In two brothers affected by the disease, no *SOD1* abnormality could be found (Robberecht et al., 1997).

Genetics and SALS

A genetic basis at least contributing to the pathogenesis of SALS is suspected. Some genes underlying the disease in a small subset of SALS patients or representing a risk factor for SALS have been reported.

SOD1 mutations and SALS

Several groups have investigated whether *SOD1* abnormalities could be involved in the pathogenesis of SALS. In each of these studies, some 'sporadic' patients with exonic *SOD1* mutations have been identified. Their number varies from 3 to 7% (reviewed in (Andersen, 2001)). Some mutations have even been found in isolated cases only. Some of these patients should be considered 'apparently' sporadic, as their family history is often incomplete or paternity not proven. In addition, the parents may be too young or may have died at too young an age to be sure that they will not be or would not have been affected (see below).

Because of the clinical similarity between *SOD1*-FALS and SALS, some authors have suggested SALS to be secondary to somatic mutations of *SOD1* in (motor) neurons, but no evidence for such mutations has been found so far (Shaw et al., 1997). Others have suggested SALS to be caused by non-mutational modifications of SOD1 (Bredesen et al., 1997). Abnormal posttranslational changes (glycation, carbonylation, mixed disulphide formation) have been hypothesized to induce the same gain of function as mutations do. No evidence in support of this hypothesis has been presented so far.

Neurofilament genes and SALS

Transgenic mice overexpressing the heavy (Cote et al., 1993) or light (Xu et al., 1993) subunit of neurofilament develop a selective motor neuron atrophy or degeneration. Furthermore, neuropathologists have always drawn attention to neurofilamentous swellings (spheroids) in ALS motor neuron bodies and proximal axons. Therefore, a role for neurofilaments in the pathogenesis of ALS has often been considered. In 5 unrelated SALS patients, Figlewicz et al., (Figlewicz et al., 1994) identified mutations in the heavy subunit of neurofilaments (NF-H). All mutations were localised in the KSP repeat domain of the protein. This domain in the C-terminal region of the protein is crucial for neurofilament assembly, crosslinking, and phosphorylation. Surprisingly, four patients had the same 3 bp deletion, while the fifth patient had a 102-bp deletion. All patients were heterozygous for the mutation. In another 351 patients (and 306 controls), no deletions were present. Al-Chalabi et al. (Al-Chalabi et al., 1999) studied 530 patients and found deletions in the KSP domain of NF-H in three SALS and one FALS patients, while a 84-bp deletion was reported in one patient by Tomkins et al., (Tomkins et al., 1998). Disappointingly, two other studies on SALS and FALS patients failed to identify any abnormality in the gene encoding NF-H or the other NF subunits (Rooke et al., 1996; Vechio et al., 1996). The occurrence of NF-H mutations in ALS is thus extremely rare (10 patients in almost a thousand screened), but the role of neurofilaments in ALS remains of major interest. Studies of mutant *SOD1* mice have shown that eliminating NF-L expression in these mice (Williamson et al., 1998) or increasing NF-L or NF-H expression (Couillard-Despres et al., 1998, 2000; Kong and Xu, 2000) prolongs the life span of these animals. These findings await further clarification.

SALS and glutamate transporters

The possible involvement of excitotoxicity in the pathogenesis of ALS is discussed by Shaw and Kuncl in Chapter 3. Pertinent to the genetics of ALS is the finding of a mutation in the EAAT2 gene in an isolated SALS patient. Loss of the EAAT2 (GLT-1) protein in SALS patients has been reported by the Kuncl and Rothstein laboratory (Rothstein et al., 1995; Rothstein et al., 1995). The mechanism explaining this loss remains uncertain. Aberrant mRNA processing has been suggested by some (Lin et al., 1998), but denied by other researchers using more substantial controls (Meyer et al., 1999; Honig et al., 2000). No exonic mutations in the glial or neuronal glutamate transporters have been identified in SALS or FALS (Bristol & Rothstein 1996; Meyer et al., 1998; Aoki et al., 1998). In one out of 200 SALS a basepair change was found (Aoki et al., 1998). This mutation results in the substitution of a glycosylated arginine residue by a cysteine residue at position 211 of the EAAT2 sequence. The loss of a glycosylation site results in the impairment of the intracellular trafficking of the protein. Surface expression of the transporter and thus glutamate transport capacity is reduced (Trotti et al., 2001). Possibly, this results in insufficient clearance of glutamate from the intercellular space and excitotoxicity.

Other genes underlying SALS

Isolated cases have been reported with a mutation in the cytochrome c oxidase subunit I gene (Comi et al., 1998) or in the APEX nuclease gene (Olkowski et al., 1998; Hayward et al., 1999). The significance of these findings remains uncertain.

Genetic risk factors for SALS

As the ε4 allele of the *apoE* gene is considered to be a risk factor for the development of Alzheimer's disease, it may be speculated that *apoE* is also involved in the pathogenesis of other neurodegenerative diseases such as ALS. Different groups have investigated the distribution of the *apoE* alleles in the ALS population. They found contradictory results. Al-Chalabi et al. (Al-Chalabi et al., 1996) and Moulard et al. (Moulard et al., 1996) found the ε4 allele to be over-represented in bulbar-onset ALS patients. However, several other groups could not detect any effect of the *apoE* alleles on the age of onset, site of onset, or duration of disease (Mui et al., 1995; Smith et al., 1996; Siddique et al., 1998b; Thijs et al., 2000; Bachus et al., 1997; Drory et al., 2001). If one pools all studies, no significant association can be found (n = 1117; χ^2-test: p>0.5). One group noted the ε4 allele to be a poor prognostic factor (Drory et al., 2001). For the time being, it seems fair to say that the role of *apoE* in the pathogenesis of ALS is probably limited.

The *SMN* gene product is an attractive candidate to play a role in the motor neuron degeneration of ALS. Moulard et al., (Moulard et al., 1998) found an unusually high number of deletions of the centromeric version of the *SMN* gene (*SMN2*) in patients with a rapidly progressive lower motor neuron syndrome. Others found *SMN2* deletions to be more frequent in SALS with both upper and lower motor neuron findings (Veldink et al., 2001). The authors suggest that these deletions may act as a susceptibility factor. A similar effect has been suggested for the *LIF* gene (Giess et al., 2000). Although *SMN1* deletions are not found in SALS (Moulard et al., 1998; Veldink et al., 2001), an abnormal copy number of the *SMN1* gene, the gene which is deleted in SMA, may be a susceptibility factor for SALS (Corcia et al., 2002). Further studies are needed to test these highly interesting hypotheses.

Clinical use of the SOD1 mutational analysis

SOD1 mutations are easy to detect: most laboratories use SSCP and direct sequencing. However, caution is needed when a mutation analysis is performed in the clinical setting. The medical, psychological and ethical implications of the identification of a mutation causing a disease such as ALS deserve major attention. Discussions on the use of presymptomatic tests in autosomal dominant, late-onset neurodegenerative diseases are difficult to summarize. Most authors strongly recommend following the guidelines developed for Huntington's disease (Research Group on Huntington's Chorea, 1994). Only a few issues will be discussed here in view of the specific problems in ALS.

Detection of mutations in ALS patients

When an ALS patient reports a family history of ALS, a critical approach is needed and confirmation should be sought in medical records. Patients and doctors confuse the long list of conditions that impair ambulation or speech, especially when occuring in elderly patients. On the other hand, when no relatives are known to be affected, one needs to assess whether the family history is reliable. Some patients are not well enough informed about their family to allow conclusions. It is crucial to establish the age of the parents alive or at time of death. One should not jump to conclusions when a patient's parents are younger than 70 years or died before age 70 of a condition different from ALS.

When autosomal dominant transmission is identified in a pedigree, a careful approach is needed. A full explanation of the implications needs to be provided to the patient. These implications are often not fully realized by the patient and his/her relatives, even though they come up with the history themselves. Even when patients and relatives know a disease to occur in the family, they do not always logically link this to risk for transmission to off-spring. It often requires a long discussion with the patient to help him or her to decide whether, when and how his/her relatives are to be informed about the familial nature of the disease.

If it is still unknown whether a patient's FALS is *SOD1*-associated or not, it should be explained to the patient that for some forms a test is available; time should be taken to explain both the implications of such test and its lack of implications. It should be made clear that the mutational analysis has no clear advantages for the patient personally. There is no evidence that a therapy other than the one recommended for SALS should be initiated (see below). One should avoid inducing false expectations.

In four out of five families, FALS is not *SOD1*-associated and no mutations will be found. If so, it should be made clear to the patient that this does not imply that the disease is not familial! However obvious this might seem, it is not always clear to those not familiar with the test, including patients, relatives and doctors.

If an *SOD1* mutation is identified, it may be tempting to use antioxidants as a treatment for *SOD1*-FALS patients, because of the evidence for oxidative stress in the pathogenesis mentioned above. However, although vitamin E and selenium delay the onset of disease in transgenic *SOD1* mice (Gurney et al., 1996), there is no evidence that antioxidants delay disease progression in animals or in humans. The results from the *SOD1* mutational analysis, therefore, do not really influence management of the patient. Although some mutations are statistically associated with certain clinical characteristics, we consider intra- and interfamilial variability large enough to not use these data in a clinical setting. We think that for all these reasons, the patient should be clearly informed about what the test actually teaches and what it does not teach, to avoid unrealistic expectations.

Some centers perform *SOD1* mutational analyses in all SALS patients, because, as mentioned, some SALS patients will be found to carry *SOD1* mutations and thus will be only 'apparently' sporadic. We have abandoned that policy because it creates confusion for patients, has low yield, and is quite expensive. If the family history is truly negative, we consider the case as sporadic and do not perform genetic tests. However, if a patient's family history is not complete or reliable, or if the age of the patient's parents does not allow us to exclude familial occurrence, we are cautious, and will perform the *SOD1* mutational analysis if indicated.

Presymptomatic diagnosis – preclinical testing

The clinically non-affected family members of a FALS patient should first be informed whether a test is available or not. This means that in at least one affected member of that family an *SOD1* mutation must have been identified. This is not always the case as no affected patient may be alive. Sometimes one can try to retrieve DNA from biopsy or autopsy specimens, etc. One should be cautious when performing an *SOD1* mutational analysis in an asymptomatic person in whose family association with the *SOD1* gene has not been demonstrated, as a negative result (absence of mutations) in this individual might induce a false sense of 'safety'.

When the affected relative has *SOD1*-associated ALS, a cautious approach to the individuals at risk is highly recommended. We follow virtually completely the guidelines that are used for Huntington's disease (Research Group on Huntington's Chorea, 1994). General guidelines suggest that only individuals aged 18 or older be tested, and that the question should always come from the individual at risk him/herself and not from any other person (parents, children, spouse). Careful and professional assessment of the motivation of an individual, his or her expectations, and his or her ability to cope should be performed before obtaining the sample. Results of tests performed in a research setting should never be used in a clinical setting.

In a first visit of an asymptomatic person at risk for *SOD1*-FALS, we concentrate on extensively informing them about the implications (or lack of implications) of the test. In a second round, the patient is tested neurologically, psychiatrically, and socially. The neurology consult is considered essential, because it is commonly accepted that the patient should be 'free of disease' or else the test is not a 'preclinical' test. Admittedly, even if an asymptomatic patient has some subtle clinical or electromyographic abnormalities (which could be the first signs of ALS), we consider the procedure as a preclinical one. It is best to offer asymptomatic patients with signs of initial disease the same support as those who do not yet show these signs (yet). A psychiatric consultation will assess the motivation of the patient and explore the risks of the test. The social consultation will assess the supports that are available to the patient. When the patient has gone through these stages, we rediscuss the test during the next visit and, if the patient wants to continue, we obtain a blood sample and perform the test. The results will be discussed during several visits thereafter, while a dense web of medical, psychological and social support is provided for the patient.

Problems arise when one leaves this well-defined pathway. Some individuals at risk ask the results only to be announced when negative, which is of course impossible. Some patients refuse to go through the whole procedure and 'want the results of *their* blood test'. Although understandable, we do not follow that line of thought, because one might harm a patient by providing information she/he is unable to use or deal with. Some doctors want to know whether an individual carries a mutation to 'better interpret the complaints' of a patient. We adhere to the rule that only the individual can ask for the test.

Sometimes, the result of a test for one individual automatically yields a result for another one who may not want to have that information, as shown in Figure 4.4. The 27-year old woman (III.3), mother of three children, wants to know whether she is a carrier or not, while her mother (II.3) definitely does not want to know. In such instances, priorities can be difficult to identify.

A major ethical issue arises when an individual carrying an *SOD1* mutation requests prenatal diagnosis and, if the unborn child carries the mutation,

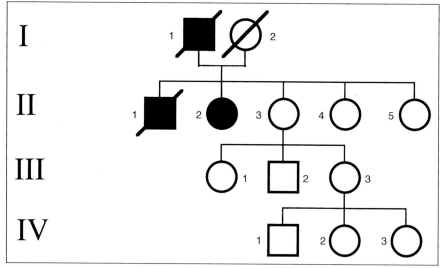

Fig. 4.4 Hypothetical FALS pedigree. Preclinical testing for individual III.3 may provide unwanted information for relative II.3

requests abortion. Similarly, ethical issues arise when a couple requires selective *in vitro* fertilization to avoid birth of an individual carrying the mutation. This issue is the object of a difficult ethical debate, that should take many scientific, medical, social, and psychological concepts into account.

References

Aguirre T, Van Den Bosch L, Goetschalckx K, et al. (1998) Increased sensitivity of fibroblasts from ALS patients to oxidative stress. Ann Neurol 43: 452–457.

Al-Chalabi A, Andersen PM, Nilsson P, et al. (1999) Deletions of the heavy neurofilament subunit tail in amyotrophic lateral sclerosis. Hum Mol Genet 8: 157–64.

Al-Chalabi A, Andersen PM, Shaw PC, et al. (1998) Recessive amyotrophic lateral sclerosis families with the D90A SOD1 mutation share a common founder: evidence for a linked protective disorder. (submitted)

Andersen PM (1997) Amyotrophic lateral sclerosis and CuZn-superoxide dismutase. Umea University Medical Dissertation, Department of Clinical Neurosciences and Clinical Chemistry, University of Umea.

Andersen PM, Nilsson P, Ala-Murula et al. (1995) Amyotrophic lateral sclerosis associated with homozygosity for an Asp90A1a mutation in CuZn-superoxide dismutase. Nature Genet 10: 61–66.

Andersen PM, Forsgren L, Binzer M, et al. (1996) Autosomal recessive adult-onset amyotrophic lateral sclerosis associated with homozygosity for Asp90 Ala CuZn-superoxide dismutase mutations. A clinical and genealogical study of 36 patients. Brain 119: 1153–1172.

Andersen PM, Nilsson P, Keränen ML, et al. (1997) Phenotypic heterogeneity in motor neuron disease patients with CuZn-superoxide dismutase mutations in Scandinavia. Brain 120: 1723–1737.

Andersen PM. (2000) Genetic factors in the early diagnosis of ALS. Amyotroph Lateral Scler Other Motor Neuron Disord 1 Suppl 1: S31–42.

Andersen PM. (2001) Genetics of sporadic ALS. Amyotroph Lateral Scler Other Motor Neuron Disord 2 Suppl 1: S37–41.

Andrus PK, Fleck TJ, Gurney ME, Hall ED. (1998) Protein oxidative damage in a transgenic mouse model of familial amyotrophic lateral sclerosis. J Neurochem 71: 2041–8.

Aoki M, Ogasawara M, Matsubara Y, et al. (1993) Mild ALS in Japan associated with novel SOD mutation. Nature Genet 5: 323–324.

Aoki M, Ogasawara M, Matsubara Y, et al. (1994) Familial amyotrophic lateral sclerosis in Japan associated with H46R mutation in CuZn superoxide dismutase gene: a possible new subtype of familial ALS. J Neurol Sci 126: 77–83.

Aoki M, Abe K, Houi K, et al. (1995) Variance of age at onset in a Japanese family with amyotrophic lateral sclerosis associated with a novel Cu/Zn superoxide dismutase mutation. Ann Neurol 37: 676–679.

Aoki M, Lin C, Rothstein JD, et al. (1998) Mutations in the glutamate transporter EAAT2 gene do not cause abnormal EAAT2 transcripts in amyotrophic lateral sclerosis. Ann Neurol 43: 645–653.

Bachus R, Bader S, Gessner R, et al. (1997) Lack of association of apolipoprotein E epsilon 4 allele with bulbar-onset motor neuron disease. Ann Neurol 41: 417.

Beal MF, Ferrante RJ, Browne SE, et al. (1997) Increased 3-nitrotyrosine in both sporadic and familial amyotrophic lateral sclerosis. Ann Neurol 42: 644–654.

Beckman JS, Larson M, Smith CE, et al. (1993) ALS, SOD and peroxynitrite. Nature 364: 584.

Bendotti C, Prosperini E, Kurosaki M, et al. (1997) Selective localization of mouse aldehyde oxidase mRNA in the choroid plexus and motor neurons. Neuroreport 8: 2343–2349.

Bereznai B, Winkler A, Borasio GD, et al. (1997) A novel SOD1 mutation in an Austrian family with amyothrophic lateral sclerosis. Neuromuscul Disord 7: 113–116.

Bobowick AR, Brody JA (1973) Epidemiology of motor-neuron diseases. N Eng J Med 288: 1047–1055.

Bogdanov MB, Ramos LE, Xu Z, Beal MF. (1998) Elevated "hydroxyl radical" generation in vivo in an animal model of amyotrophic lateral sclerosis. J Neurochem 71: 1321–4.

Borchelt DR, Wong PC, Becher MW, et al. (1998) Axonal transport of mutant superoxide dismutase 1 and focal axonal abnormalities in the proximal axons of transgenic mice. Neurobiol Dis 5: 27–35.

Bowling AC, Schulz JB, Brown RH, Jr., Beal MF. (1993) Superoxide dismutase activity, oxidative damage, and mitochondrial energy metabolism in familial and sporadic amyotrophic lateral sclerosis. J Neurochem 61: 2322–5.

Bowling AC, Barkowski EE, McKenna Yasek D, et al. (1995) Superoxide dismutase concentration and activity in familial amyotrophic lateral sclerosis. J Neurochem 64: 2366–2369.

Bredesen DE, Ellerby LM, Hart PJ, et al. (1997) Do posttranslational modifications of CuZnSOD lead to sporadic amyotrophic lateral sclerosis? Ann Neurol 42: 135–138.

Bristol LA, Rothstein JD (1996) Glutamate transporter gene expression in amyotrophic lateral sclerosis motor cortex. Ann Neurol 39: 676–679.

Brown Jr RH, Robberecht W. (2001) Amyotrophic Lateral Sclerosis: Pathogenesis. Seminars in Neurology 21: 131–139.

Bruening W, Roy J, Giasson B, Figlewicz DA, Mushynski WE, Durham HD. (1999) Up-regulation of protein chaperones preserves viability of cells expressing toxic Cu/Zn-superoxide dismutase mutants associated with amyotrophic lateral sclerosis. J Neurochem 72: 693–9.

Bruijn LI, Beal MF, Becher MW, et al. (1997) Elevated free nitrotyrosine levels, but not proteinbound nitrotyrosine or hydroxyl radicals, throughout amyotrophic lateral sclerosis (ALS)-like disease implicate tyrosine nitration as an aberrant in vivo property of one familial ALS-linked superoxide dismutase 1 mutant. Proc Natl Acad Sci USA 94: 7606–7611.

Bruijn LI, Houseweart MK, Kato S, et al. (1998) Aggregation and motor neuron toxicity of an ALS-linked SOD1 mutant independent from wild-type SOD1. Science 281: 1851–4.

Calder VL, Domigan NM, George PM, et al. (1995) Superoxide dismutase (glu100gly) in a family with inherited motor neuron disease: detection of mutant superoxide dismutase activity and the presence of heterodimers. Neurosci Lett 189: 143–146.

Chance PF, Rabin BA, Ryan SG, et al. (1998) Linkage of the gene for an autosomal dominant form of juvenile amyotrophic lateral sclerosis to chromosome 9q34. Am J Hum Genet 62: 633–640.

Cleveland DW, Rothstein JD. (2001) From charcot to lou gehrig: deciphering selective motor neuron death in ALS. Nat Rev Neurosci 2: 806–19.

Comi GP, Bordoni A, Salani S, et al. (1998) Cytochrome c oxidase subunit I microdeletion in a patient with motor neuron disease. Ann Neurol 43: 110–6.

Cote F, Collard JF, Julien JP. (1993) Progressive neuronopathy in transgenic mice expressing the human neurofilament heavy gene: a mouse model of amyotrophic lateral sclerosis. Cell 73: 35–46.

Couillard-Despres S, Zhu Q, Wong PC, Price DL, Cleveland DW, Julien JP. (1998) Protective effect of neurofilament heavy gene overexpression in motor neuron disease induced by mutant superoxide dismutase. Proc Natl Acad Sci U S A 95: 9626–30.

Couillard-Despres S, Meier J, Julien JP. (2000) Extra axonal neurofilaments do not exacerbate disease caused by mutant Cu, Zn superoxide dismutase. Neurobiol Dis 7: 462–70.

Crow JP, Sampson JB, Zhuang Y, et al. (1997) Decreased zinc affinity of amyotrophic lateral sclerosis-associated superoxide dismutase mutants leads to enhanced catalysis of tyrosine nitration by peroxynitrite. J Neurochem 69: 1936–1944.

Cudkowicz ME, McKenna-Yasek D, Sapp PE, et al. (1997) Epidemiology of mutations in superoxide dismutase in amyotrophic lateral sclerosis. Ann Neurol 41: 210–221.

Cudkowicz MR, McKenna-Yasek D, Chen C, et al. (1998) Limited corticospinal tract involvement in amyotrophic lateral sclerosis subjects with the A4V mutation in the copper/zinc superoxide dismutase gene. Ann Neurol 43: 703–710.

Deng H-X, Hentati A, Tainer JA, et al. (1993) Amyotrophic lateral sclerosis and structural defects in CuZn superoxide dismutase. Science 261: 986–989.

Deng H-X, Tainer JA, Mitsumoto H, et al. (1995) Two novel SOD1 mutations in patients with familial amyotrophic lateral sclerosis. Hum Mol Genet 4: 1113–1116.

Drory VE, Birnbaum M, Korcyzn AD, Chapman J. (2001) Association of APOE varepsilon4 allele with survival in amyotrophic lateral sclerosis. J Neurol Sci 190: 17–20.

Durham HD, Roy J, Dong L, et al. (1997) Aggregation of mutant Cu/Zn superoxide dismutase proteins in a culture model of ALS. J Neuropathol Exp Neurol 56: 523–530.

Ellerby LM, Cabelli DE, Graden JA, et al. (1996) Copper-zinc superoxide dismutase: why not pH-dependent? J Am Chem Soc 118: 6556–6561.

Elshafey A, Lanyon WG, Connor JM (1994) Identification of a new missense mutation in exon 4 of the Cu/Zn superoxide dismutase (SOD-1) gene in a family with amyotrophic lateral sclerosis. Hum Mol Genet 3: 363–364.

Enayat ZE, Orrell RW, Claus A, et al. (1995) Two novel mutations in the gene for copper zinc superoxide dismutase in UK families with amyotrophic lateral sclerosis. Hum Mol Genet 4: 1239–1240.

Esteban J, Rosen DR, Bowling AC, et al. (1994) Identification of two novel mutations and a new polymorphism in the gene for Cu/Zn superoxide dismutase in patients with amyotrophic lateral sclerosis. Hum Mol Genet 3: 997–998.

Estevez AG, Crow JP, Sampson JB, et al. (1999) Induction of nitric oxide-dependent apoptosis in motor neurons by zinc-deficient superoxide dismutase. Science 286: 2498–500.

Eyer J, Cleveland DW, Wong PC, Peterson AC (1998) Pathogenesis of two axonopathies does not require axonal neurofilaments. Nature 391: 584–587.

Ferrante RJ, Browne SE, Shinobu LA, et al. (1997) Evidence of increased oxidative damage in both sporadic and familial amyotrophic lateral sclerosis. J Neurochem 69: 2064–2074.

Figlewicz DA, Krizus A, Martinoli MG, et al. (1994) Variants of the heavy neurofilament subunit are associated with the development of amyotrophic lateral sclerosis. Hum Mol Genet 3: 1757–1761.

Fridovich I (1986) Superoxide dismutases. Adv Enzymol 58: 61–97.

Getzoff ED, Tainer JA, Stempien MM, et al. (1989) Evolution of CuZn superoxide dismutase and the greek key ß-barrel structural motif. Proteins 5: 322–336.

Giess R, Beck M, Goetz R, Nitsch RM, Toyka KV, Sendtner M. (2000) Potential role of LIF as a modifier gene in the pathogenesis of amyotrophic lateral sclerosis. Neurology 54: 1003–5.

Graham AJ, Macdonald AM, Hawkes CH (1997) British motor neuron disease twin study. J Neurol Neurosurg Psychiatry 62: 562–569.

Gurney ME, Pu H, Chiu AY, et al. (1994) Motor neuron degeneration in mice that express a human Cu, Zn Superoxide Dismutase Mutation. Science 64: 1772–1775.

Gurney ME, Cutting FB, Zhai P, et al. (1996) Benefit of vitamin E, riluzole, and gabapentin in a transgenic model of familial amyotrophic lateral sclerosis. Ann Neurol 39: 147–157.

Hadano S, Hand CK, Osuga H, et al. (2001) A gene encoding a putative GTPase regulator is mutated in familial amyotrophic lateral sclerosis 2. Nat Genet 29: 166–73.

Hall ED, Andrus PK, Oostveen JA, Fleck TJ, Gurney ME. (1998) Relationship of oxygen radical-induced lipid peroxidative damage to disease onset and progression in a transgenic model of familial ALS. J Neurosci Res 53: 66–77.

Hamida MB, Hentati F, Hamida CB (1990) Hereditary motor system diseases (chronic juvenile amyotrophic lateral sclerosis). Brain 113: 347–363.

Hand CK, Mayeux-Portas V, Khoris J, et al. (2001) Compound heterozygous D90A and D96N SOD1 mutations in a recessive amyotrophic lateral sclerosis family. Ann Neurol 49: 267–71.

Hand CK, Khoris J, Salachas F, et al. (2002) A Novel Locus for Familial Amyotrophic Lateral Sclerosis, on Chromosome 18q. Am J Hum Genet 70: 251–256.

Hansen C, Gredal O, Werdelin L, et al. (1998) A 4-bp insertion in the CuZn-superoxide dismutase gene associated with familial amyotrophic lateral sclerosis. Hum Mutat (In press.)

Haverkamp LJ, Appel V, Appel SH (1995) Natural history of amyotrophic lateral sclerosis in a database population. Brain 118: 707–719.

Hawkes CH, Graham AJ (1992) National UK motor neuron disease twin study using the death discordant approach. Ann Neurol 32: 272–273.

Hayward C, Colville S, Swingler RJ, Brock DJ. (1999) Molecular genetic analysis of the APEX nuclease gene in amyotrophic lateral sclerosis. Neurology 52: 1899–901.

Hentati A, Bejaoui K, Pericak-Vance MA, et al. (1994) Linkage of recessive familial amyotrophic lateral sclerosis to chromosome 2q33-q35. Nature Genet 7: 425–428.

Hentati A, Ouahchi K, Pericak-Vance MA, et al. (1997) Linkage of a common locus for recessive amyotrophic lateral sclerosis. Am J Hum Genet Suppl 61: A279.

Hentati A, Ouahchi K, Pericak-Vance MA, et al. (1998) Linkage of a commoner form of recessive amyotrophic lateral sclerosis to chromosome 15q15-q22 markers. Neurogenetics 2: 55–60.

Hirano A, Kurland LT, Sayre GP (1967) Familial amyotrophic lateral sclerosis. A subgroup characterized by posterior and spinocerebellar tract involvement and hyaline inclusions in the anterior horn cells. Arch Neurol 16: 232–243.

Hirano A, Donnefeld H, Sasaki S, et al. (1984) Fine structural observations of neurofilamentous changes in amyotrophic lateral sclerosis. J Neuropathol Exp Neurol 43: 461–470.

Hirano M, Fujii J, Nagai Y, et al. (1994) A new variant Cu/Zn superoxide dismutase (Val7Æ Glu) deduced from lymphocyte mRNA sequences from Japanese patients with familial amyotrophic lateral sclerosis. Biochem Biophys Res Commun 204: 572–577.

Honig LS, Chambliss DD, Bigio EH, Carroll SL, Elliott JL. (2000) Glutamate transporter EAAT2 splice variants occur not only in ALS, but also in AD and controls. Neurology 55: 1082–8.

Hosler BA, Nicholson GA, Sapp PC, et al. (1996) Three novel mutations and two variants in the gene for Cu/Zn superoxide dismutase in familial amyotrophic lateral sclerosis. Neuromusc Disord 6: 361–366.

Hosler BA, Siddique T, Sapp PC, et al. (2000) Linkage of familial amyotrophic lateral sclerosis with frontotemporal dementia to chromosome 9q21-q22. Jama 284: 1664–9.

Hutton M, Lendon CL, Rizzu P, et al. (1998) Association of missense and 5′-splice-site mutations in tau with the inherited dementia FTDP-17. Nature 393: 702–5.

Ikeda M, Abe K, Aoki M, et al. (1995a) A novel point mutation in the Cu/Zn superoxide dismutase gene in a patient with familial amyotrophic lateral sclerosis. Hum Mol Genet 4: 491–492.

Ikeda M, Abe IK, Aoki M, et al. (1995b) Variable clinical symptoms in familial amyotrophic lateral sclerosis with a novel point mutation in the Cu/Zn superoxide dismutase gene. Neurology 45: 2038–2042.

Jackson M, Al-Chalabi A, Enayat ZE, et al. (1997) Copper/zinc superoxide dismutase 1 and sporadic amyotrophic lateral sclerosis: analysis of 155 cases and identification of a novel insertion mutation. Ann Neurol 42: 803–807.

Jones CT, Swingler RJ, Brock DJH (1994) Identification of a novel SOD1 mutation in an apparently sporadic amyotrophic lateral sclerosis patient and the detection of Ile 113Thr in three others. Hum Mol Genet 3: 649–650.

Jones CT, Swingler RJ, Simpson SA, et al. (1995) Superoxide dismutase mutations in an unselected cohort of Scottish amyotrophic lateral sclerosis patients. J Med Genet 32: 290–292.

Juneja T, Pericak-Vance MA, Laing NG, et al. (1997) Prognosis in familial amyotrophic lateral sclerosis. Neurology 48: 55–57.

Kawamata S, Shimohama S, Hasegawa H, et al. (1995) Deletion and point mutations in superoxide dismutase-1 gene in amyotrophic lateral sclerosis (abstract.). XIth TMIN International Symposium:Amyotrophic Lateral Sclerosis, Progress and Perspectives in basic research and clinical application, Tokyo.

Kawata A, Kato S, Hayashi H, et al. (1997) Prominent sensory and autonomic disturbances in familial amyotrophic lateral sclerosis with a Gly93Ser mutation in the SOD1 gene. J Neurol Sci 153: 82–85.

Kong J, Xu Z. (2000) Overexpression of neurofilament subunit NF-L and NF-H extends survival of a mouse model for amyotrophic lateral sclerosis. Neurosci Lett 281: 72–4.

Kostrzewa M, Burck-Lehman, Müller U (1994) Autosomal dominant amyotrophic lateral sclerosis: a novel mutation in the Cu/Zn superoxide dismutase-1 gene. Hum Mol Genet 3: 2261–226.

Kostrzewa M, Damian MS, Müller U (1996) Superoxide dismutase 1: identification of 4 novel mutations in a case of familial amyotrophic lateral sclerosis. Hum Genet 98: 48–50.

Kunst CB, Mezey E, Brownstein MJ, et al. (1997) Mutations in SOD1 associated with amyotrophic lateral sclerosis cause novel protein interactions. Nat Genet 15: 91–94.

Lee MK, Marszalek JR, Cleveland DW (1994) A mutant neurofilament subunit causes massive, selective motor neuron death: implications for the pathogenesis of human motor neuron disease. Neuron 13: 975–988.

Leigh PN, Dodson A, Swash M, et al. (1989) Cytoskeletal abnormalities in motor neuron disease. Brain 112: 521–535.

Levanon D, Lieman-Hurwitz J, Dafni N, et al. (1985) Architecture and anatomy of the chromosomal locus in human chromosome 21 encoding the Cu/Zn superoxide dismutase. The EMBO J 4: 77–84.

Lewis J, McGowan E, Rockwood J, et al. (2000) Neurofibrillary tangles, amyotrophy and progressive motor disturbance in mice expressing mutant (P301L) tau protein. Nat Genet 25: 402–5.

Li TM, Alberman E, Swash M (1988) Comparison of sporadic and familial disease amongst 580 cases of motor neuron disease. J Neurol Neurosurg Psychiatry 51: 778–784.

Lin G, Bristol GA, Jin L, et al. (1998) Aberrant RNA processing in a neurodegenerative disease: a common cause for loss of glutamate EAAT2 protein in sporadic amyotrophic lateral sclerosis. Neuron 16: 675–686.

Lynch T, Sano M, Marder KS, et al. (1994) Clinical characteristics of a family with chromosome 17-linked disinhibition-dementia-parkinsonism-amyotrophy complex. Neurology 44: 1878–1884.

Metcalf CW, Hirano A (1971) Amyotrophic lateral sclerosis. Clinicopathological studies of a family. Arch Neurol 24: 518–523.

Meyer T, Lenk U, Küther G, et al. (1995) Studies of the coding region of the neuronal glutamate transporter gene in amyotrophic lateral sclerosis. Ann Neurol 37: 817–819.

Meyer T, Munch C, Volkel H, Booms P, Ludolph AC. (1998) The EAAT2 (GLT-1) gene in motor neuron disease: absence of mutations in amyotrophic lateral sclerosis and a point mutation in patients with hereditary spastic paraplegia. J Neurol Neurosurg Psychiatry 65: 594–6.

Meyer T, Fromm A, Munch C, et al. (1999) The RNA of the glutamate transporter EAAT2 is variably spliced in amyotrophic lateral sclerosis and normal individuals. J Neurol Sci 170: 45–50.

Morita M, Aoki M, Abe K, et al. (1996) A novel two-base mutation in the Cu/Zn superoxide dismutase gene associated with familial amyotrophic lateral sclerosis in Japan. Neurosci Lett 205: 79–82.

Moulard B, Camu W, Brice A, et al. (1995) A previously undescribed mutation in the SOD1 gene in a French family with atypical ALS (abstract). 6th International Symposium on ALS/MND, II, Dublin, Ireland, 22.

Moulard B, Sefiani A, Laamri A, et al. (1996) Apolipoprotein E genotyping in sporadic amyotrophic lateral sclerosis: evidence for a major influence on the clinical presentation and prognosis. J Neurol Sci 139: 34–37.

Moulard B, Salachas F, Chassande B, et al. (1998) Association between centromeric deletions of the SMN gene and sporadic adult-onset lower motor neuron disease. Ann Neurol 43: 640–644.

Mui S, Reveck GW, Mc Kenna-Yasek D, et al. (1995) Apolipoprotein E epsilon 4 allele is not associated with earlier age at onset in amyotrophic lateral sclerosis. Ann Neurol 38: 460–463.

Mulder DW, Kurland LT, Offord KP, et al. (1986) Familial adult motor neuron disease: amyotrophic lateral sclerosis. Neurology 36: 511–517.

Nakano R, Sato S, Inuzuka T, et al. (1994) A novel mutation in Cu/Zn superoxide dismutase gene in Japanese familial amyotrophic lateral sclerosis. Bichem Biophys Res Commun 200: 695–703.

Nakashima K, Watanabe Y, Kuno N, et al. (1995) Ahnormality of Cu/Zn superoxide dismutase (SOD1) activity in Japanese familial amyotrophic lateral sclerosis with two base pair deletion in tbe SOD1 gene. Neurology 45: 1019–1020.

Olkowski ZL. (1998) Mutant AP endonuclease in patients with amyotrophic lateral sclerosis. Neuroreport 9: 239–42.

Orrell R, de Belleroche J, Marklund S, et al. (1995a) A novel SOD mutant and ALS. Nature 374: 504–505.

Orrell RW, King AW, Hilton DA, et al. (1995b) Familial amyotrophic lateral sclerosis with a point mutation of SOD1: intrafamilial heterogeneity of disease duration associated with neurofibrillary tangles. J Neurol Neurosurg Psychiatry 59: 266–270.

Orrell RW, Habgood JJ, Gardiner I, et al. (1997a) Clinical and functional investigation of 10 missense mutations and a novel frameshift insertion mutation of the gene for copper-zinc superoxide dismutase in UK families with amyotrophic lateral sclerosis. Neurology 48: 746–751.

Orrell RW, Habgood JJ, Shepherd DI, et al. (1997b) A novel mutation of SOD-1 (Gly108Val) in familial amyotrophic lateral sclerosis. Eur J Neurol 4: 48–51.

Pedersen WA, Fu W, Keller JN, et al. (1998) Protein modification by the lipid peroxidation product 4-hydroxynonenal in the spinal cords of amyotrophic lateral sclerosis patients. Ann Neurol 44: 819–24.

Pramatarova A, Goto S, Nanba E, et al. (1994) A two basepair deletion in the SOD1 gene causes familial amyotrophic lateral sclerosis. Hum Mol Genet 3: 2061–2062.

Pramatarova A, Figlewicz DA, Krizus A, et al. (1995) Identification of new mutations in the Cu/Zn superoxide dismutase gene of patients with familial amyotrophic lateral sclerosis. Am J Hum Genet 56: 592–596.

Rabin BA, Griffin JW, Crain BJ, Scavina M, Chance PF, Cornblath DR. (1999) Autosomal dominant juvenile amyotrophic lateral sclerosis. Brain 122: 1539–50.

Radunovic A, Leigh PN (1996) Cu/Zn superoxide dismutase gene mutations in amyotrophic lateral sclerosis: correlation between genotype and clinical features. J Neurol Neurosurg Psych 61: 565–572.

Reaume AG, Elliott JL, Hoffman EK, et al. (1996) Motor neurons in Cu/Zn superoxide dismutase-deficient mice develop normally but exhibit enhanced cell death after axonal injury. Nat Genet 13: 43–7.

Research Group on Huntington's Chorea (1994) Guidelines for the molecular genetics predictive test in Huntington's disease. Neurology 44: 1533–1536.

Ripps ME, Huntley GW, Hof PR, Morrison JH, Gordon JW. (1995) Transgenic mice expressing an altered murine superoxide dismutase gene provide an animal model of amyotrophic lateral sclerosis. Proc Natl Acad Sci U S A 92: 689–93.

Robberecht W, Sapp P, Viaene MK, et al. (1994) Cu/Zn superoxide dismutase activity in familial and sporadic amyotrophic lateral sclerosis. J Neurochem 62: 384–387.

Robberecht W, Aguirre T, Van Den Bosch L, et al. (1996a) D90A heterozygosity in the SOD1 gene is associated with familial and apparently sporadic amyotrophic lateral sclerosis. Neurology 47: 1336–1339.

Robberecht W, Vermylen P, Theys P, et al. (1996b) ApoE and SMN genotypes in amyotrophic lateral sclerosis. International Motor Neuron Disease Association. Chicago 1996.

Robberecht W, Aguirre T, Van Den Bosch L, et al. (1997) Familial juvenile focal amyotrophy of the upper extremity (Hirayama disease). Arch Neurol 54: 46–50.

Robberecht W. (2000) Oxidative stress in amyotrophic lateral sclerosis. J Neurol 247 Suppl 1: 11–6.

Rooke K, Figlewicz DA, Han FY, Rouleau GA. (1996) Analysis of the KSP repeat of the neurofilament heavy subunit in familiar amyotrophic lateral sclerosis. Neurology 46: 789–90.

Rosen DR, Siddique T, Patterson D, et al. (1993) Mutations in Cu/Zn superoxide dismutase gene are associated with familial amyotrophic lateral sclerosis. Nature 362: 59–62.

Rosen DR, Bowling AC, Patterson D, et al. (1994) A frequent ala 4 to val superoxide dismutase-1 mutation is associated with rapidly progressive familial amyotrophic lateral sclerosis. Hum Molec Genet 3: 981–987.

Rothstein JD, Martin LJ, Kuncl RW (1992) Decreased glutamate transport by the brain and spinal cord in amyotrophic lateral sclerosis. N Engl J Med 326: 1464–1468.

Rothstein JD, Van Kammen M, Levey AI, Martin LJ, Kuncl RW. (1995) Selective loss of glial glutamate transporter GLT-1 in amyotrophic lateral sclerosis. Ann Neurol 38: 73–84.

Rouleau GA, Clark K, Pramatarova A, et al. (1996) SOD1 mutations is associated with accumulation of neurofilaments in amyotrophic lateral sclerosis. Ann Neurol 39: 128–131.

Sapp PC, Rosen DR, Hosler BA, et al. (1995) Identification of three novel mutations in the gene for Cu/Zn superoxide dismutase in patients with familial ayotrophic lateral sclerosis. Neuromuscul Disord 5: 353–357.

Shaw PJ, Ince PG, Falkous G, Mantle D. (1995) Oxidative damage to protein in sporadic motor neuron disease spinal cord. Ann Neurol 38: 691–5.

Shaw CE, Enayat ZE, Powell JF, et al. (1997a) Familial amyotrophic lateral sclerosis: molecular pathology of a patient with a SOD1 mutation. Neurology 49: 1612–1616.

Shaw PJ, Tomkins J, Slade JY, et al. (1997b) CNS tissue Cu/Zn superoxide dismutase (SOD1) mutations in motor neuron disease (MND). Neuroreport 8: 3923–3927.

Shaw CE, Enayat ZE, Chioza BA, et al. (1998) Mutations in all five exons of SOD-1 may cause ALS. Ann Neurol 43: 390–394.

Shibata N, Hiranao A, Kobayashi M, et al. (1996) Intense superoxide dismutase-1 immunoreactivity in intracytoplasmic hyaline inclusions of familial amyotrophic lateral sclerosis with posterior column involvement. J Neuropathol Exp Neurol 55: 481–490.

Siddique T (1991a) Molecular genetics of familial amyotrophic lateral sclerosis. Adv Neurol 56: 227–231.

Siddique T, Deng HX (1996) Genetics of amyotrophic lateral sclerosis. Hum Mol Gen 5: 1465–1470.

Siddique T, Figlewicz DA, Pericak-Vance MA, et al. (1991) Linkage of a gene causing familial amyotrophic lateral sclerosis to chromosome 21 and evidence of genetic-locus heterogeneity. N Engl J Med 324: 1381–1384.

Siddique T, Hong S, Brooks B, et al. (1998a) X-linked dominant locus for late-onset familial amyotrophic lateral sclerosis. Am J Hum Genet 63: A308.

Siddique T, Pericak-Vance MA, Caliendo J, et al. (1998b) Lack of association between apolipoprotein E genotype and sporadic amyotrophic lateral sclerosis. Neurogenetics 1: 213–6.

Singh RJ, Karoui H, Gunther MR, et al. (1998) Reexamination of the mechanism of hydroxyl radical adducts formed from the reaction between familial amyotrophic lateral sclerosis-associated Cu, Zn superoxide dismutase mutants. Proc Natl Acad Sci USA 95: 6675–6680.

Själander A, Beckman G, Deng HX, et al. (1995) The D90 A mutation results in a polymorphism of Cu, Zn superoxide dismutase that is prevalent in northern Sweden and Finland. Hum Mol Genet 4: 1105–1108.

Smith RG, Haverkamp LJ, Case S, et al. (1996) Apolipoprotein E epsilon 4 in bulbar-onset motor neuron disease. Lancet 348: 334–335.

Spillantini MG, Goedert M. (1998) Tau protein pathology in neurodegenerative diseases. Trends Neurosci 21: 428–33.

Spittaels K, Van den Haute C, Van Dorpe J, et al. (1999) Prominent axonopathy in the brain and spinal cord of transgenic mice overexpressing four-repeat human tau protein. Am J Pathol 155: 2153–65.

Strong MJ, Hudson AJ, Alvord WG. (1991) Familial amyotrophic lateral sclerosis, 1850–1989: a statistical analysis of the world literature. Can J Neurol Sci 18: 45–58.

Suthers G, Laing N, Wilton S, et al. (1994) 'Sporadic' motoneuron disease due to familial SOD1 mutation with low penetrance. Lancet 344: 1773.

Thijs V, Peeters E, Theys P, Matthijs G, Robberecht W. (2000) Demographic characteristics and prognosis in a Flemish amyotrophic lateral sclerosis population. Acta Neurol Belg 100: 84–90.

Tomkins J, Usher P, Slade JY, et al. (1998) Novel insertion in the KSP region of the neurofilament heavy gene in amyotrophic lateral sclerosis (ALS). Neuroreport 9: 3967–70.

Trotti D, Rolfs A, Danbolt NC, Brown RH, Jr., Hediger MA. (1999) SOD1 mutants linked to amyotrophic lateral sclerosis selectively inactivate a glial glutamate transporter. Nat Neurosci 2: 427–33.

Trotti D, Aoki M, Pasinelli P, et al. (2001) Amyotrophic lateral sclerosis-linked glutamate transporter mutant has impaired glutamate clearance capacity. J Biol Chem 276: 576–82.

Vanopdenbosch L, Robberecht W. (2001) Unusual phenotype with the G93C mutation in SOD1 in familial ALS. Neurology 56: A445.

Vechio JD, Bruijn LI, Xu Z, et al. (1996) Sequence variants in human neurofilament proteins: absence of linkage to familial amyotrophic lateral sclerosis. Ann Neurol 40: 603–610.

Veldink JH, van den Berg LH, Cobben JM, et al. (2001) Homozygous deletion of the survival motor neuron 2 gene is a prognostic factor in sporadic ALS. Neurology 56: 749–52.

Veltema AN, Ross RAC, Bruyn GW (1990) Autosomal dominant adult amyotrophic lateral sclerosis: a six-generation Dutch family. J Neurol Sci 97: 93–115.

Vernant JC, Cabre P, Smadja D, et al. (1997) Recurrent optic neuromyelitis with endocrinopathies: a new syndrome. Neurology 48: 58–64.

Watanabe M, Aoki M, Abe K, et al. (1997) A novel missense point mutation (S134N) of the Cu/Zn superoxide dismutase gene in a patient with familial motor neuron disease. Hum Mutat 9: 69–71.

Wiedau-Pazos MW, Goto JJ, Rabizadeh S, et al. (1996) Altered reactivity of superoxide dismutase in familial amyotrophic lateral sclerosis. Science 271: 515–518.

Wilhelmsen KC, Lynch T, Pavlou E, et al. (1994) Localization of disinhibition-dementia-Parkinsonism–amyotrophy complex to 17q21–22. Am J Hum Genet 55: 1159–1165.

Williamson TL, Bruijn LI, Zhu Q, et al. (1998) Absence of neurofilaments reduces the selective vulnerability of motor neurons and slows disease caused by a familial amyotrophic lateral sclerosis-linked superoxide dismutase 1 mutant. Proc Natl Acad Sci U S A 95: 9631–6.

Williamson TL, Cleveland DW. (1999) Slowing of axonal transport is a very early event in the toxicity of ALS-linked SOD1 mutants to motor neurons. Nat Neurosci 2: 50–6.

Wong PC, Pardo CA, Borchelt DR, et al. (1995) An adverse property of a familial ALS-linked SOD1 mutation causes motor neuron disease characterized by vacuolar degeneration of mitochondria. Neuron 14: 1105–16.

Wright RM, Weigel LK, VarellaGarcia M, et al. (1997) Molecular cloning, refined chromosomal mapping and structural analysis of the human gene encoding aldehyde oxidase (AOX1), a candidate for the ALS2 gene. Redox-Report 3: 135–144.

Xu Z, Cork LC, Griffin JW, Cleveland DW. (1993) Increased expression of neurofilament subunit NF-L produces morphological alternations that resemble the pathology of human motor neuron disease. Cell 73: 23–33.

Yang Y, Hentati A, Deng HX, et al. (2001) The gene encoding alsin, a protein with three guanine-nucleotide exchange factor domains, is mutated in a form of recessive amyotrophic lateral sclerosis. Nat Genet 29: 160–5.

Yim MB, Kang J-H, Yim H-S, Kwak HS, et al. (1996) A gain-of-function of an amyotrophic lateral sclerosis-associated Cu, Zn-superoxide dismutase mutant: an enhancement of free radial formation due to a decrease in k_m for hydrogen peroside. Proc Natl Acad Sci USA 93: 5709–5714.

Yim HS, Kang JH, Chock PB, Stadtman ER, Yim MB. (1997) A familial amyotrophic lateral sclerosis-associated A4V Cu, Zn-superoxide dismutase mutant has a lower Km for hydrogen peroxide. Correlation between clinical severity and the Km value. J Biol Chem 272: 8861–3.

Yulug IG, Katsanis N, de Belleroche J, et al. (1995) Am improved protocol for the analysis of SOD1 gene mutations and a new mutation in exon 4. Hum Mol Genet 4: 1474.

Zu JS, Deng HX, Lo TP, et al. (1997) Exon5 encoded domain is not required for the toxic function of mutant SOD1 but essential for the dismutase activity: identification and characterization of two new SOD1 mutations assiociated with familial amyotrophic lateral sclerosis. Neurogenetics 1: 65–71.

CHAPTER 5

Spinal muscular atrophy

Thomas O. Crawford

Now in its second century, research into the devastating childhood genetic disorder spinal muscular atrophy (SMA) has entered a new age. In the first 100 years after Werdnig described the disorder in 1891, SMA research was dominated by clinical description and nosologic debate between lumpers and splitters, who differed over whether the spectrum of the disorder consisted of one or many separate, but similar, diseases. With localization of the gene to chromosome 5q13 (Brzustowicz et al., 1990; Gilliam et al., 1990), the nosologic issue was resolved in favor of the lumpers: SMA is a single disease that manifests over a range of severity. Of greater importance, however, is that identification of the pathogenic survival motor neurone (*SMN*) gene (Lefebvre et al., 1995) generated a number of high quality questions about the molecular genetics, molecular biology, and cell biology of SMN and the pathophysiology of SMA. We now have realistic grounds for hope that the answers to these questions will establish a basis for therapy.

SMA is perhaps the most common serious autosomal recessive disorder of children worldwide, affecting children on all continents in roughly equal proportions (Emery, 1991). This contrasts to the other, better known, genetic recessive disorders of children, cystic fibrosis and sickle cell anemia, which are each largely restricted to a single race. Approximately 1 in 6000 children have SMA, ranging in severity from a fatal disorder to one of mild weakness. The separation of SMA into three separate groups based upon severity of weakness continues to have value for purposes of clinical description.

- SMA 1, or Werdnig–Hoffmann disease, is defined by weakness manifest before 6 months of age and the inability to maintain a sitting position at any time in life.
- A more mildly affected group, defined by inability to stand, is known as SMA 2.
- SMA 3, or Kugelberg–Welander disease, describes those individuals with SMA and weakness who are nonetheless able to stand and walk.

Clinical aspects

Diagnostic features

The hallmark of the clinical presentation is diffuse weakness due to denervation of muscle. Generally the legs are affected more than arms, and the limbs are affected more than cranial muscles; hence the designation 'spinal'. Formal clinical criteria for the diagnosis, formulated by an international consortium in 1990 (Munsat, 1991), include the requirements that:

1 Weakness be symmetric and affect trunk muscles as well as limb muscles, with proximal more than distal weakness.
2 Denervation be demonstrated by both electrophysiologic and biopsy features.
3 Any other CNS involvement, serious impairment of other organ systems, arthrogryposis, sensory loss, or eye or facial muscle weakness exclude the diagnosis.

While these criteria were important to define unambiguous cases in the early 1990s when diagnostic certainty was important to linkage analysis, subsequent development of a 'gold standard' genetic test for the diagnosis utilizing *SMN* has led to the realization that many of these original exclusionary clinical criteria were too restrictive. SMA is now recognized as responsible for a broader phenotype. Among the most seriously affected are infants with congenital arthrogryposis and widespread CNS neuropathologic changes (Devriendt et al., 1997). At the other end of the spectrum are adults with EMG and biopsy features of denervation but who are fully strong (Brahe et al., 1995; Hahnen et al., 1995; Wang et al., 1996; Bussaglia et al., 1997).

The features of typical Werdnig–Hoffmann disease are sufficiently distinctive to experienced observers that the physical exam alone can be both very sensitive and specific for the diagnosis. Affected infants have a bright and active face and eyes that are highly communicative. Weakness of intercostal muscles and relative sparing of the diaphragm produces a paradoxic breathing pattern, characterized by depression of the ribcage during inspiration. Later in the course of the disease, the chest assumes the shape of a bell, as intercostal weakness leads to collapse of the upper chest while the relatively powerful diaphragm pulls the lowest ribs upward, producing an outward flair. At rest, the tongue often trembles spontaneously along its surface, but this sign, which has been much emphasized, may have poor specificity in practice, given an overall tendency of normal infants' tongues to tremble while disturbed. Infants with Werdnig–Hoffmann disease can often move their toes and fingers but are generally unable to raise outstretched limbs against gravity. With time, bulbar muscles become weaker, and affected infants develop difficulty with sucking, swallowing, and crying, and eventually difficulty with maintaining the airway.

Children with milder forms of SMA will generally not manifest weakness of the intercostal muscles but do have the same caudal to rostral distribution of weakness. In many, the foot has a pes planus deformity identified by calcaneal valgus, eversion of the forefoot and collapse of the arch. The outstretched hand and fingers often manifest a fine tremor, termed minipolymyoclonus, which is merely a reflection of coarsened motor control that results from fewer motor units each having a greater size (Moosa and Dubowitz, 1973). Deep tendon reflexes are lost or diminished commensurate with the loss of muscle power.

Laboratory features

Motor nerve conduction studies have normal conduction velocity for age if the compound muscle action potential is high enough to be easily measured; it is often, however, quite low. Sensory nerve studies are normal. Infants with severe SMA tend to have abundant abnormal spontaneous activity on EMG. Voluntary motor unit recruitment is reduced, but most if not all of the remaining motor unit potentials are normal in duration or even of short duration. EMG of more mildly affected individuals demonstrates reduced recruitment of voluntary motor units, but differs from that of more severely affected infants by the paucity of abnormal spontaneous activity and the large amplitude and prolonged duration of the surviving voluntary motor units (Hausmanowa-Petrusewicz, 1988; Crawford et al., 1995). Serum creatine kinase activity is often mildly elevated, especially in the mildest cases (Rudnik-Schöneborn et al., 1998).

Muscle biopsy demonstrates two populations of muscle fibers (Dubowitz, 1995). In the more severely weakened child there are vast numbers of tiny denervated muscle fibers demonstrating both type I and type II histochemical features and a second population of normal to very large fibers, generally displaying type I histochemical features. This is a rare instance where type I fibers are pathologically enlarged in caliber. Widespread muscle fiber atrophy will increase the ratio of connective to contractile tissue, but this proportionate increase is not a measure of ongoing connective tissue proliferation. Muscle spindles are abundant for the same reason. The architecture within fibers is not disrupted, although occasional rods can be seen, a feature that is common in denervated muscle (Konno et al., 1987). In younger, more severely affected infants the enlarged fibers appear to congregate in regions due to severe atrophy of the intermixed denervated fibers. The presence of intercalated severely atrophic fibers within a region partially supplied by an intact motor neuron, yet absence of fiber type grouping, suggests that the capacity for sprouting is limited in severely affected young patients. In contrast, older and stronger patients with SMA have significant fiber type grouping, indicating that chronic reinnervation of adjacent denervated muscle fibers proceeds unhindered.

In the last few years the clinical indications for EMG and muscle biopsy have diminished dramatically, particularly in patients with highly characteristic clinical features, because of the high sensitivity and specificity of the *SMN* gene test (see below).

Clinical course and pathophysiologic implications

The outcome of SMA depends greatly upon the severity of weakness. Infants with SMA 1 generally have very limited survival, with 75% and 95% mortality by the first and second birthdays, respectively (Ignatius, 1994; Thomas and

Dubowitz, 1994, Zerres et al., 1997). Such infants inevitably develop respiratory insufficiency. During upper respiratory illnesses, diminished clearance of airway secretions and progressive atelectasis often prove fatal. Those with milder forms of SMA survive longer. The lifespan of individuals with type 3 SMA is unknown, but can be near normal, while that of individuals with type 2 SMA is variable, linked closely to the severity of weakness and the vigor of palliative treatment.

In all forms of SMA, however, the clinical course is unusual for a degenerative disease. Affected individuals tend to have the greatest rate of loss of muscle power at the outset; over time, residual muscle power stabilizes and may cease to change. There are striking examples of individuals with stable yet profoundly diminished power that is maintained over years or even decades (Dubowitz, 1964, 1995). This is in marked contrast to the apparent linear decline of amyotrophic lateral sclerosis (Chapter 1). An important distinction, however, is that functional abilities decline (Russman et al., 1996) more than muscle power (Russman et al., 1992). Increases in weight, size, or deformity may compromise function even while power measured in a gravity neutral plane remains unchanged. This tendency for increasing stability over time is characteristic of all forms of the disorder, though a caveat applies to infants with severe weakness. In these infants different regions of the body may behave as if they are at different stages of this 'front loaded' degenerative course: at the time of diagnosis chest and bulbar innervated muscles may be near normal but thereafter weaken further, while the limbs which are already enfeebled at the time of diagnosis maintain about the same amount of profoundly diminished power over time.

A biologic explanation for this unusual clinical course is not immediately apparent. It seems likely that motor neurons are lost more rapidly at the outset of the disease than later in the course. How this unusual kinetics of neuronal loss could be regulated is at best speculative. One attractive hypothesis is that the neurodegeneration is related, in some fashion, to a defect in developmental apoptosis. During normal development, an initial excess of motor neurons is cut back to the appropriate size by programmed cell death. This may represent insufficient trophic support from the available muscle to these 'extra' motor neurons, a process which eventually matches the number of surviving motor neurons to the mass of muscle tissue to be innervated. The kinetics of cell loss due to SMA appears to be similar to this developmental process; in each circumstance surviving neurons become increasingly resistant to degeneration. A second hypothesis is that motor neurons naturally vary in some characteristic that determines vulnerability to degeneration. Finally, it is possible that survival itself confers an advantage for further survival. One could imagine that the increases in motor unit size that accompany neighboring denervation permit access to an increased supply of a trophic support derived from muscle. Against this latter hypothesis, however, is the lack of correlation of neuronal survival to the differences in motor unit size that are manifest naturally in different muscles.

As noted, loss of functional abilities may not parallel change in muscle power, which appears to be more stable over time. There are several possible explanations for this discrepancy.

First, children with significant weakness are at substantial risk for complications such as scoliosis or obesity, which increase the amount of muscle power necessary to maintain a stable level of function. These complications are often treatable or preventable, and thus should be a major focus of therapy (see below).

Second, the meaning of stable strength in a developing and growing child is not clear. Given a stable (small) number of functioning youthful motor units, each with an expanded motor unit territory of hypertrophic muscle fibers, should we expect increasing power proportionate to growth of the limbs, or should power remain constant?

Finally, experience with postpolio amyotrophy suggests that neurons innervating an enlarged complement of muscle fibers may encounter special difficulties over time. Late losses of muscle power could be due to pruning of overextended motor units by a similar age-related mechanism that is only indirectly related to the initial pathogenesis of SMA.

Neuropathology of SMA

The dominant neuropathology of SMA is the paucity of motor neurons in the anterior horn of the spinal cord (reviewed in Crawford and Pardo, 1996). Most of the remaining motor neurons appear normal, but a small number display chromatolytic changes, with swelling of the perikaryon, margination of the nucleus, and dispersion of the clumped RNA within the cytoplasm. It is not known if these chromatolytic, ballooned neurons are in a prolonged agonal state or are successfully reacting to an unknown stress. Though initially thought to be restricted to motor neurons, careful pathologic studies on a small number of severely affected infants indicates that motor neurons are only the most vulnerable of a number of different neuronal populations, the commonality of which is not clear. In these infants with an early demise, chromatolytic cells can be found in the ventrolateral thalamus, mesencephalic nucleus, pallidum, nucleus basalis of Meynert, brainstem motor nuclei, and to a lesser degree in more widespread areas (Towfighi et al., 1985; Bingham et al., 1997; Bürglen et al., 1997; Devriendt et al., 1997).

Genetics of SMA

The gene for SMA was among the last of the common genetic disorders to be identified by classical genetics, largely because the SMA-critical region of chromosome 5q is marked by substantial heterogeneity in the normal population (Campbell et al., 1997; Chen et al., 1998). Within this region multiple defined markers differ in copy number, to the frustration of a large international effort (reviewed in Crawford, 1996). Moreover, the SMA-critical region is notably unstable in multiple different cloning vectors (Thompson et al., 1995) and during human meiosis (Melki et al., 1994; Campbell et al., 1997; Wirth et al., 1997). This finding is probably responsible for the high and apparently near uniform incidence of SMA world-wide, since there appears to be a stable production of new mutant alleles. In 1995, the SMA-critical region was found to consist of a large inverted duplication, each portion of which contains near-homologous copies of the genes *p44* (Bürglen et al., 1997), neuronal apopto-sis inhibitory protein (*NAIP*) (Burghes 1997), and *SMN* (Lefebvre et al., 1995) (Figure 5.1). The tight association of SMA to deletion (Lefebvre et al., 1995) and disabling intragenic mutations (for review, Lefebvre et al., 1998) of the telomeric copy of *SMN*, *SMN1*, identify it as the pathogenic gene responsible for SMA.*

Genetic diagnosis

By conservative estimates, 95% of all cases of SMA are associated with homozygous absence of the *SMN1* sequence (Lefebvre et al., 1995). As such, the genetic test for *SMN1* surpasses EMG and muscle biopsy as the most sen-sitive confirmatory test for the disorder once clinical suspicion is raised. Genetic testing can be done easily with PCR techniques (van der Steege et al., 1995) and is offered in many accredited diagnostic genetic laboratories.

A few patients remain who have classical clinical features of the disease without homozygous loss of *SMN1*. While some of these patients have a sep-arate but similar phenocopy disorder (Zerres et al., 1995; Velasco et al., 1996; Parsons et al., 1998a), others have true SMA and the normal *SMN* gene test is falsely reassuring. In these patients an intragenic mutation of *SMN1* disrupts *SMN* translation or SMN function, but the remaining DNA sequence of exons 7 and 8 are of correct size and are amplified normally on the standard PCR-based test. One way of identifying which patients have such an occult muta-tion of *SMN*, and which have an SMA-phenocopy disorder uses a newly developed semi-quantitative PCR technique that can determine *SMN1* and *SMN2* copy number (McAndrew et al., 1997). By Bayesian analysis, a child with characteristic clinical features of SMA and a single copy of *SMN1* is far more likely to have an unrecognized intragenic mutation in this single copy than to be both a genetic carrier for SMA and suffer from a different SMA-phenocopy neuromuscular disease. If a patient has classic clinical, electrodi-agnostic and pathologic features of SMA, evaluation of *SMN1* copy number can determine those cases with a reduced copy number of *SMN1* in whom sequencing would likely demonstrate a disabling mutation (Parsons et al., 1998b).

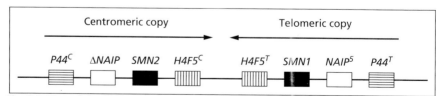

Fig. 5.1 Map of the SMA critical region of chromosome 5q13. Each of the *SMN1* neighboring genes have at least one homolog in a large duplicated segment lying just centromeric to the parent region

SMN1 is also known as SMN^T and SMN_{TEL}, and *SMN2* as SMN^C and SMN_{CEN}

The specificity of the *SMN* gene test for SMA appears to be very high because homozygous deletion of *SMN1* has not been identified in the general population. In a few families where the proband is affected by mild SMA, a sibling or parent also has a homozygous deletion of *SMN1* but does not manifest clinical weakness (Brahe et al., 1995; Hahnen et al., 1995; Wang et al., 1996; Bussaglia et al., 1997). Whether these individuals (some of whom have signs of chronic denervation on EMG) are presymptomatic or will remain asymptomatic through life, is unknowable at present. For the diagnosis of symptomatic individuals, however, false-positive diagnosis of SMA with an abnormal *SMN1* gene test is highly unlikely.

One unresolved feature of the genetics of SMA is that homozygous deletion of *SMN1* is characteristic of all three clinical forms of the disorder. Differences in phenotype thus cannot be related to the loss of *SMN1* itself. At present, genetic techniques are unable to predict phenotype severity. Fortunately, this issue is rarely important in clinical practice, as the test is now generally applied to diagnosis of weak children, in whom the phenotype is already apparent, or to the prospective diagnosis of fetal siblings, who if affected are strongly inclined to manifest weakness similar to the proband.

Molecular genetics of *SMN* and genotype/phenotype correlations

There is a complex interrelationship between *SMN1* and *SMN2* at two different levels – the gene and the gene product – each of which is critical to both the existence of the disorder and the severity of its expression. The coding sequences of these two genes are virtually identical, differing in only two base pairs within exons 7 and 8. Two forms of mutations appear to be responsible for the bulk of pathogenic *SMN* alleles. The first is a deletion event, removing *SMN1* and possibly its neighboring genes *NAIP*, *p44* or *H4F5*. The other is a 'conversion' mutation in which the telomeric copy, *SMN1*, is converted to the centromeric sequence in both exons 7 and 8 together (Burghes 1997; Campbell et al., 1997) or, less often, only exon 7 (Hahnen et al., 1996; DiDonato et al., 1997). Gene conversion, first well studied in yeast, involves the nonreciprocal modification of near-homologous sequences that are generally in close proximity (Liskay et al., 1987). Conversion mutations are responsible for an increasing number of human genetic disorders, now including congenital adrenal hyperplasia (Higashi et al., 1988), neurofibromatosis (Hulsebos et al., 1996), von Willebrand's disease (Eikenboom et al., 1994) and polycystic kidney disease (Watnick et al., 1998). Of these two most common forms of *SMN1* mutations, deletion is more often associated with a severe phenotype, where conversion is usually associated with milder disease expression.

Both genes produce an identical protein product (Lefebvre et al., 1995). The exon 8 sequence difference is in the 3' untranslated region while the exon 7 difference is synonymous, producing a different codon for the same amino acid. The promoter region has not been compared carefully, but transcript from each gene can be found in equal abundance in all tissues measured. Although they are similar at the level of translation, promotion, and predicted protein product, *SMN1* and *SMN2* differ substantially at the level of posttranslational modification. *SMN1* produces a full length protein, whereas most *SMN2* transcript is cleaved in exon 7 (*SMN Δ7*) with only minor production of full length protein.

Homozygous deletion of *SMN2* is found in approximately 5% of normal individuals, but surprisingly there are no known cases of patients with homozygous loss of both *SMN1* and *SMN2*. The presumption, borne out by experience in the knockout of the single *SMN* gene in mice (Schrank et al., 1997), is that loss of both *SMN1* and *SMN2* is an early embryonic lethal trait.

Because disease in affected siblings is usually similar in severity (Pearn, 1980; Zerres et al., 1997), and because all forms of SMA share the common loss of *SMN1*, phenotype severity must be related to another genetic element that is tightly linked to *SMN1*. Two non-exclusive general hypotheses have been offered as explanations. First is the possibility that deletion of *SMN1* also removes a neighboring gene that modifies expression of the disease. The adjacent localization of genes that are genetically distinct but related by cellular function has a precedent in the association of the gene for vesicular acetylcholine transport protein with that for the synthetic enzyme choline acetyltransferase (Erickson et al., 1994). Candidate genes for this modifying role based upon their location next to *SMN1* are *NAIP* (Rodrigues et al., 1996; Wang et al., 1997), *p44* (Carter et al., 1997), or *H4F5* (Scharf et al., 1998). In the case of *NAIP*, the contiguous gene hypothesis is enhanced by biologic plausibility. *NAIP* (for neuronal apoptosis inhibitory protein) is so named because of its homology to baculovirus anti-apoptotic genes (Roy et al., 1995). Enhancement of *NAIP* expression reduces neuronal cell death from ischemia (Xu et al., 1997a), and *NAIP* is abundantly expressed in rat in all of the neuronal cell populations that are known to be vulnerable in severe forms of SMA (Xu et al., 1997b). However, both the absence and the presence of *NAIP* can occur across the spectrum of SMA. The argument for importance of the nuclear transcription subunit factor *p44* is less compelling. Homozygous deletion of *p44* is less frequent and less well correlated with severity than is *NAIP*. Finally, *H4F5* is the closest gene to *SMN*, with its deletion having the best correlation to phenotype, but differences between the telomeric and centromeric forms have not been identified and its function is unknown (Scharf et al., 1998).

The alternative hypothesis, that *SMN2* is the major modifier of SMA phenotype, has been gaining acceptance from a variety of different lines of evidence. With some notable exceptions, copy number of *SMN2* correlates with milder phenotype (Velasco et al., 1996; Burghes 1997; Campbell et al., 1997; Simard et al., 1997; Parsons et al., 1998a). The above argument for neighboring genes can also be said to support *SMN2* as the modifying gene, as deletion of *SMN1* (associated with severe SMA) decreases by one the number of total copies of *SMN1* and *SMN2*, while conversion mutation (associated with milder SMA) increases by one the copy number of *SMN2*. Indeed, among patients with an intact copy of *NAIP*, *SMN2* copy number correlates well with phenotype across the spectrum of disease, suggesting that *NAIP*-intact patients with severe disease nonetheless have a small deletion mutation of *SMN1* (Taylor et al., 1998). The number of copies of the human *SMN2* gene added to a mouse model of SMA missing the native *SMN* gene is correlated with severity of weakness and duration of survival (Monani et al., 2000). An important final argument for *SMN2* as the main regulator of phenotype expression is that it produces a small amount of the full length SMN protein. This supports the idea that *SMN2* gene copy number can mitigate loss of the major full length SMN producer, *SMN1*, to the extent that an increase in copy number produces a commensurate increase in full length *SMN* transcripts and protein synthesis. For all of these reasons it appears that *SMN2* is the leading candidate for the phenotype modifier gene. It is critical to the occurrence and probably to the expression of SMA. In the setting of homozygous loss of *SMN1*, absence of *SMN2* is lethal in early embryogenesis, but increasing copy number preserves motor neuron numbers in a graded way from severe to inconsequential manifestation.

The biology of SMN

SMN is widely expressed in all tissues, but immunocytochemical studies show abundant staining in particular within the cytoplasm of fetal motor neurons (Lefebvre et al., 1997). SMN is also localized in small nuclear structures, termed 'gems', that are similar in size and shape, and maintain close proximity, to nuclear coiled bodies (Liu and Dreyfuss, 1996). The number of immunolabeled gems correlates inversely with phenotype severity (Coovert et al., 1997) as does protein level in lymphoblasts and in a limited number of fetal spinal cord specimens (Lefebvre et al., 1997).

When first identified, the sequence of *SMN* generated no immediate hypothesis about function since there was no homology to any known gene or gene product. However, a laboratory investigating RNA processing proteins had previously pulled the then-anonymous *SMN* transcript out of a human library by the yeast two-hybrid system (Liu and Dreyfuss, 1996). It is now clear that at least one function of SMN is to aid in the assembly of spliceosomal small nuclear ribonucleoprotein (snRNP) complexes in the cytoplasm (Figure 5.2) (Mattaj 1998). SMN is tightly associated with SMN interacting protein (SIP1), which in turn is essential to assembly of spliceosomal Sm proteins and small nuclear RNAs (snRNA) exported from the nucleus into an snRNP complex. This complex then re-enters the nucleus to process newly transcribed pre-mRNA into mature mRNA (Liu et al., 1997; Fischer et al., 1997). SMN not only aids in the cytoplasmic assembly of the snRNP complex but also has additional nuclear functions for pre-mRNA splicing. It appears to be necessary to recycling or regeneration of snRNPs within the nucleus, possibly through its association with the gem bodies to maintain ongoing splicing function (Pellizzoni et al., 1998).

Most of the rare *SMN* missense mutations probably work as recessives, failing to perform this vital function in snRNP biogenesis and regeneration. The possibility exists, however, that some mutations of *SMN* may act as dominant negatives, disrupting snRNP function in a manner similar to that of a laboratory generated partial SMN protein (Pellizzoni et al., 1998). SMN has a self-binding, or oligomerization, domain in exon 6, where most of the known missense mutations of *SMN* reside (Lefebvre et al., 1995; Hahnen et al., 1997; McAndrew et al., 1997; Talbot et al., 1997). Efficiency of oligomerization correlates well with phenotype severity among these individuals, and SMNΔ7 fails

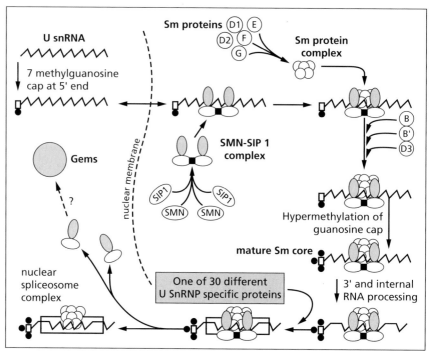

Fig. 5.2 The role of SMN in the cytoplasmic assembly of the spliceosomal complex. One of five U snRNAs (U1, U2, U5 or a complex of U4 and U6) are methylated at the 5' guanosine before bidirectional export to the cytoplasm where it binds to the assembled SMN-SIP1 complex. A preformed complex of five Sm proteins and three additional single Sm proteins are added. The 5' guanosine is then hypermethylated to produce the mature SnRNP spliceosomal core. The U snRNA is then processed internally and cleaved at the 3' end, and an additional catalytic protein, specific to each initial U snRNA, is added as the complex is imported into the nucleus. The SMN-SIP 1 complex is removed either before or with nuclear importation; how SMN and SIP1 enter the nucleus to inhabit nuclear gems is unknown

to oligomerize, suggesting that SMN self-association is important to pathogenesis (Lorson et al., 1998). *SMN* also has a nucleic acid binding domain in exon 2 that is also impaired by the exon 6 missense mutations, suggesting that oligomerization stabilizes RNA binding and further highlighting its role in pre-mRNA splicing (Lorson and Androphy 1998) (Figure 5.3).

Given this fundamental housekeeping function in pre-mRNA processing, it is easy to understand why complete loss of SMN is an early embryonic lethal. Why motor neurons are particularly vulnerable to diminished capacity for pre-mRNA splicing is unknown, though it is clear that they are highly synthetic neurons, producing a large volume of neurofilament protein daily for maintenance of their large axonal caliber through slow axonal transport.

Another possible function of SMN has been suggested for which the connection to excessive neuronal loss may be more easily understood. Co-expression of SMN with Bcl-2 confers a synergistic effect against various apoptotic challenges that is not present in the absence of Bcl-2. Moreover, *SMNΔ7* and one of the known missense SMN proteins failed to demonstrate this effect.

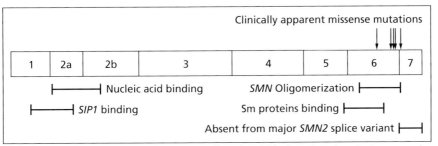

Fig. 5.3 Map of the *SMN* transcript. Known functional binding domains cluster around exons 2 and 6, in regions of high sequence conservation. The known clinically apparent missense mutations also cluster around exon 6, including one that lies within the exon 7 region that is lost in the major splice variant produced by *SMN2*

This finding, if confirmed, would indicate that absence of SMN is responsible for excessive apoptosis within motor neurons (Iwahahi et al., 1997).

Finally, a non-neuronal function for SMN is suggested by the finding that infants with severe SMA, but not older children or those with more mild forms of the disease, have a distinctive abnormality in fatty acid metabolism evident in plasma and fasting urine samples (Crawford et al., 1999). Because the severity of the abnormality correlates with deletion of *NAIP*, it may be due to either *SMN1* or a neighboring gene, for all of the above reasons. No single known defect in the metabolism of fatty acids can explain these findings, suggesting that the defect is due to a coordinated disruption of fatty acid metabolism at multiple sites (Crawford et al., 1999).

Treatment

There is as yet no specific treatment for SMA. However, the peculiar clinical course of SMA, in which the rate of progression diminishes with the passage of time, makes this a disease in which supportive care can have a major impact on quality and quantity of life. Complications of weakness, such as weight gain, scoliosis, or contractures, rather than continued loss of strength itself, may result in functional losses over time. Many of these complications can be partially or fully ameliorated with careful prospective treatment. Whether a portion of the functional decline experienced over many years is in fact due to a primary degeneration associated with SMA is unknown.

Orthopedic management

Orthopedic issues are of paramount importance, as weakness precipitates deformity, which in turn renders weakened muscles mechanically disadvantaged. The most important deformity is scoliosis, which often presents in individuals with type 2 SMA during the early years of rapid growth. Treatment with an external hard thoraco-lumbar-sacral orthosis (TLSO) is most successful in slowing progression when applied early while the curve is still mild, but it is uncomfortable, restricts chest wall movement and sometimes other functions, and needs to be adjusted frequently for growth. Nonetheless, treatment with a TLSO is in many circumstances capable of minimizing progression of the curve until children attain more skeletal maturity and operative spinal fusion becomes possible. Internal fixation of the spine too early, when there is still significant growth potential, may result in later deformities around the fixation. Vertical growth of the anterior portions of vertebral bodies is restrained by fixation of the posterior elements, leading to severe lordotic or torsional deformity. In light of this problem, it is generally better to try to temporize with the TLSO until growth is nearly complete. If successful, such bracing retards the scoliosis until an age when it is possible to achieve a nearly straight spine with posterior rod placement and segmental instrumentation only. The goal is to avoid the need for the much more extensive and difficult combined anterior–posterior approach to scoliosis repair, either to mobilize a severe fixed scoliotic deformity or to remove vertebral growth plates to prevent future deformity when posterior elements are fused before skeletal maturity.

Physiotherapy and adaptive aids

Treatment of limb deformities involves the same tense balance between the present and future as immediate discomfort and restricted function are exchanged for maintenance of normal anatomy and maximizing function over time. Stretching exercises, bracing, and operative interventions are most justified in individuals in whom the limb is presently functional or nearly so. Painful, risky, or time consuming therapy and operative procedures for only cosmetic purposes may be less appropriate; they signal a distortion of priorities. Such interventions come at the cost of time for normal development, education, and family life, against which the burdens and benefits should be weighed. In general, knowledge that many children with SMA have a prolonged course should be an incentive to treat potential deformities early and vigorously.

For children who can walk easily the most common problem is a progressive pes planus foot with midfoot collapse, which can lead to ankle and arch pain that limits walking. In those with difficulty walking or standing, knee and hip contractures frequently develop, placing an additional mechanical burden on maintaining an upright posture and eventually making independent standing impossible. In weaker children who are in wheelchairs full time, hip and knee contractures can, when severe, limit the ability to turn in bed, thus necessitating assistance throughout the night.

Contractures are also common in the upper extremity in children whose weakness restricts full active range of movement. Contracture progression can be retarded by frequent and regular passive stretching exercises, though for many these procedures may be uncomfortable. In general, daytime bracing restricts function. Nighttime bracing is usually only successful at slowing additional deformity. There are many individual variations, but the most common problems of the upper extremity include restricted forearm supination (with or without dislocation of the radial head), contracture of deep finger flexors restricting the hand from opening with the wrist in neutral position, and ulnar deviation of the hand at the wrist.

Pulmonary management

Pulmonary issues are most critical in those children at the severe end of the SMA spectrum. Infants with SMA have a mechanical disadvantage of the chest wall, which collapses with diaphragmatic contraction, diminishing inspiratory volume. Treatment of these very feeble infants involves early treatment of upper respiratory infections with postural drainage and percussion, antibiotics, and aerosolized bronchodilators. Infants are often more able to breathe in Trendelenberg position while lying prone or on one side, because the chest wall collapses less, diaphragmatic movement is increased as the relaxed diaphragm pushes further up into the chest, and airway secretions are more able to drain. Unfortunately, over time most infants are unable to withstand repeated pulmonary infections, as decreasing respiratory muscle power and increasing lung stiffness compromise breathing further. Families must then face difficult choices of quality versus quantity of life, as mechanical ventilation can prolong life indefinitely but at the cost of extreme dependence for all vital and nonvital functions. These issues are best addressed prospectively, though not necessarily at the time of diagnosis.

Children with moderate weakness also often have significant pulmonary problems. Nighttime assessment of sleep efficiency by continuous end-tidal CO_2 measurements and monitoring the sleep state is the best measure of incipient pulmonary insufficiency when it is not obvious in daytime functioning or pulmonary function tests. Particularly poignant is the toddler or young child with lymphoid hypertrophy and obstructive sleep apnea who recovers significant muscle power after adenotonsilectomy. For those children with marginal respiratory reserve manifest at night, or both day and night, mechanical assistance in breathing may have a very positive effect on quality and quantity of life. In many patients, assistance at night only, either with invasive or newly developing noninvasive techniques, leads to improved sleep efficiency and substantial improvements in muscle power and overall well-being.

The metabolic problems of low muscle mass

Muscle is a storage organ. Children with profoundly diminished muscle mass may face severe challenges for fuel homeostasis, leading to occult but important physiologic distortions. Limited muscle mass cannot supply energy for gluconeogenesis after calories from a meal are exhausted but before the induction of systemic lipolysis. In general, it is best to minimize fasting by using small frequent meals or continuous nighttime feeding. One must assure adequate caloric supplies by parenteral means during gastrointestinal vomiting or other catabolic challenges. Muscle is also the major store of intracellular salts and minerals, which can be lost during diarrheal illness. Children with severe reduction of muscle mass are thus at risk for the sudden onset of symptomatic hypokalemia when losses into the gastrointestinal lumen exceed whole body supply.

So far, the known details of SMN function do not predict any specific therapy. The facts that *SMN2* produces a full length SMN protein and that the truncated protein synthesized from *SMNΔ7* has not demonstrated any dominant negative effect lead naturally to the possibility that a therapy could involve upregulation of *SMN2* gene expression and transcription. Efforts to discover more about gene regulation are ongoing, as is a search for agents that might increase gene translation. If the analogy to developmental apoptosis is biologically relevant, one can hypothesize that there might be a role for trophic compounds involved in the regulation of normal motor neuron survival during development. Long after development, neurotrophic factors may enhance motor neuron survival (see Chapter 6). One important caveat for therapy comes from the clinical course of SMA: it is likely that therapy directed at rescue of motor neurons will need to be initiated early in the course of the disease to have the most effect. This subject is discussed in more detail in Chapter 9.

Ethical concerns and difficult decisions

In medicine there are few greater dilemmas than those in which surrogates must base their decision upon the perception of quality of life. These issues are even more difficult when the question concerns infants who have a long life of full self-awareness ahead of them. This dilemma arises from the need to determine whether children should be placed on life-sustaining respiratory support for acute illness or chronic respiratory insufficiency. Some infants at the most severe end of the SMA spectrum are so profoundly weak that they are never able to move or communicate in any way other than their autonomic responses. At the other end of the spectrum of SMA are individuals – who will probably never need a ventilator – who can partake in typical activities of life with minimal assistance from others. Thus, there is a continuous spectrum of morbidity from horrific to slight in SMA, and decisions about resuscitation and artificial ventilation must be made with full knowledge of this spectrum, as the following scenarios illustrate.

- Most infants with the severe Werdnig–Hoffmann form of SMA are able to communicate with their faces and to a small extent their voice, but recognizable speech is severely impaired even when they are supported until the age of language acquisition. With extensive therapy some of these infants may be fitted with microswitch devices which will support one or more dimensions of a computer mouse. Given this severe impairment of communication and the inability to manipulate the world independently without continuous support by others, most parents and care givers elect not to extend life artificially with full-time ventilation.
- Slightly stronger infants and children will be able to vocalize, support their head while sitting, and use their hands well at the time of presentation. These children have a very different ability to interact with the world. Because of the unique slow clinical course, they are generally able to continue with these skills for years (if not decades), and become able to speak understandably. Now, in the computer age, they are more able to perform typical and useful tasks independent of the need for continuous support from others. In individuals on chronic ventilator assistance the support necessary from others is proportional to their weakness. Those unable to sit independently or transfer generally require nearly full-time assistance.

There are also substantial numbers of stronger children who need respiratory support only at night. Among these patients there is little question that respiratory support, if needed, can be justified given their capacity for independent expression and action. The family and social resources that need be dedicated to their care can be considerable, however, which may raise larger and very difficult issues about resource allocation.

Since SMA manifests over a spectrum of extremes of impairment, there are patients in between for whom the issue of whether or not ventilator support can be justified is extraordinarily difficult when based upon individual quality of life, even without considering the larger family and social issues. The burdens that result from a decision to extend life by long-term ventilator support, and the benefits that arise from this support, are not equally balanced in all who are affected by the decision. Patients, parents, siblings and other family members, medical and educational communities, and society at large each have a stake in the decision, but the balance of benefits and burdens may tip in different directions. Obviously, the best decisions will be made with honest discussion amongst family members and therapists, but they will always be complicated by the multiple levels of ambiguity and disquiet among all involved, as the possibilities for remorse, guilt, impoverishment of time, marital and family discord, and sibling competition are real variables in the outcome.

One other difficult area, in many ways similar to the decision to extend life with mechanical ventilators, is the decision to terminate the pregnancy of an affected fetus. In most instances of affected sibling pairs the phenotype of the siblings will be very similar. This should provide a basis for the prospective parents to make a decision, since they are usually uniquely well informed about the burdens of the disease, having suffered with the first affected child. The ability to identify the carrier status in uncles and aunts and their spouses now raises the possibility that a fetal cousin, nephew or niece will be identified as having SMA. Decisions about continuation of the pregnancy in this circumstance may be more difficult, because the severity of the proband has less predictive value. Because one of the pathogenic alleles in the affected individual is of unknown severity, there is a wide range of phenotype severity between affected second degree relatives. The general ethics of early termination of pregnancy are, of course, beyond the scope of this chapter, but the added complexity of the fetus having a genetic disorder of unknown severity will, for some, only add more discord and pain to a difficult decision.

References

Bingham PM, Shen N, Rennert H et al. (1997) Arthrogryposis due to infantile neuronal degeneration associated with deletion of the SMNt gene. Neurology 49: 848–851.

Brahe C, Zappata S, Bertini E (1995) Presymptomatic diagnosis of spinal muscular atrophy (SMA) III confirmed by deletion analysis of the survival motor neuron gene. Am J Med Genet 59: 101–102.

Brzustowicz LM, Lehner T, Castilla LH et al. (1990) Genetic mapping of chronic childhood-onset spinal muscular atrophy to chromosome 5q11.2–13.3. Nature 344: 540–541.

Burghes AHM (1997) When is a deletion not a deletion? When it is converted. Am J Hum Genet 61: 9–15.

Bussaglia E, Tizzano EF, Illa I, Cervera C, Baiget M (1997) Cramps and minimal EMG abnormalities as preclinical manifestations of spinal muscular atrophy patients with homozygous deletions of the SMN gene. *Neurology* 48: 1443–1445.

Bürglen L, Seroz T, Miniou P, Lefebvre S et al. (1997) The gene encoding p44, a subunit of the transcription factor TFIIH, is involved in large-scale deletions associated with Werdnig-Hoffmann disease. Am J Hum Genet 60: 72–79.

Campbell L, Potter A, Ignatius J, Dubowitz V, Davies K (1997) Genomic variation and gene conversion in spinal muscular atrophy: implications for disease process and clinical phenotype. Am J Hum Genet 61: 40–50.

Carter TA, Bönnemann CG, Wang CH et al. (1997) A multicopy transcription-repair gene, BF2p44, maps to the SMA region and demonstrate SMA associated deletions. Hum Mol Genet 6: 229–236.

Chen Q, Baird SD, Mahadevan M, Besner-Johnston A et al. (1998) Sequence of a 131-kb region of 5q13.1 containing the spinal muscular atrophy candidate genes SMN and NAIP. Genomics 48: 121–127.

Coovert DD, Le TT, McAndrew PE et al. (1997) The survival motor neuron protein in spinal muscular atrophy. Hum Mol Genet 6: 1205–1214.

Crawford TO (1996) From enigmatic to problematic: the new molecular genetics of childhood spinal muscular atrophy. Neurology 46: 335–340.

Crawford TO, Pardo CA (1996) The neurobiology of childhood spinal muscular atrophy. Neurobiol Dis 3: 97–110.

Crawford TO, Chaudhry V, Sladky JT (1995) Lack of reinnervation in severe infantile spinal muscular atrophy. Ann Neurol 38:539 (Abstract).

Crawford TO, Sladky JT, Hurko O, Besner-Johnston A, Kelley RI (1999) Abnormal fatty acid metabolism in childhood spinal muscular atrophy. Ann Neurol 45: 337–343.

Devriendt K, Lammens M, Schollen E et al. (1997) Clinical and molecular genetic features of congenital spinal muscular atrophy. Ann Neurol 40: 731–738.

DiDonato CJ, Ingraham SE, Mendell JR et al. (1997) Deletion and conversion in SMA patients: Is there a relationship to severity? Ann Neurol 41: 230–237.

Dubowitz V (1964) Infantile muscular atrophy: A prospective study with particular reference to a slowly progressive variety. Brain 87: 707–718.

Dubowitz V (1995) Muscle disorders in childhood. Saunders: Philadelphia.

Eikenboom JC, Vink T, Briet E, Sixma JJ, Reitsma PH (1994) Multiple substitutions in the von Willebrand factor gene that mimic the pseudogene sequence. Proc Natl Acad Sci USA 91: 2221–2224.

Emery AEH (1991) Population frequencies of inherited neuromuscular diseases – a world summary. Neuromusc Disord 1: 19–29.

Erickson JD, Varoqui H, Schäfer MK-H et al. (1994) Functional identification of a vesicular acetylcholine transporter and its expression from a "cholinergic" gene locus. J Biol Chem 269: 21929–21932.

Fischer U, Liu Q, Dreyfuss G (1997) The SMN-SIP1 complex has an essential role in spliceosomal snlRNP biogenesis. Cell 90: 1023–1029.

Gilliam TC, Brzustowicz LM, Castilla LH et al. (1990) Genetic homogeneity between acute and chronic forms of spinal muscular atrophy. Nature 345: 823–825.

Hahnen E, Forkert R, Marke C et al. (1995) Molecular analysis of candidate genes on chromosome 5q13 in autosomal recessive spinal muscular atrophy: evidence of homozygous deletions of the SMN gene in unaffected individuals. Hum Mol Genet 4: 1927–1933.

Hahnen E, Schonling J, Rudnik-Schöneborn S, Zerres K, Wirth B (1996) Hybrid survival motor neuron genes in patients with autosomal recessive spinal muscular atrophy: new insights into molecular mechanisms responsible for the disease. Am J Hum Genet 59: 1057–1065.

Hahnen E, Schönling J, Rudnik-Schöneborn S, Raschke H, Zerres K, Wirth B (1997) Missense mutations in exon 6 of the survival motor neuron gene in patients with spinal muscular atrophy (SMA). Hum Mol Genet 6: 821–825.

Hausmanowa-Petrusewicz I (1988) Electrophysiological findings in childhood spinal muscular atrophies. Rev Neurol (Paris) 144: 716–720.

Higashi Y, Tanae A, Inoue H, Fujii-Kuriyama Y (1988) Evidence for frequent gene conversion in the steroid 21-hydroxylase P-450 (C21) gene: implications for steroid 21-hydroxylase deficiency. Am J Hum Genet 42: 17–25.

Hulsebos TJ, Bijleveld EH, Riegman PH, Smink LJ, Dunham I (1996) Identification and characterization of NF1-related loci on human chromosomes 22, 14 and 2. Hum Genet 98: 7–11.

Ignatius J (1994) The natural history of severe spinal muscular atrophy – further evidence for clinical subtypes. Neuromusc Disord 4: 527–528.

Iwahashi H, Eguhi Y, Yasuhara N, Hanafusa T, Matsuzawa Y, Tsujimoto Y (1997) Synergistic anti-apoptotic activity between Bcl-2 and SMN implicated in spinal muscular atrophy. Nature 390: 413–417.

Konno H, Iwasaki Y, Yamamoto T, Inosaka T (1987) Nemaline bodies in spinal progressive muscular atrophy: An autopsy case. Acta Neuropathol (Berl) 74: 84–88.

Lefebvre S, Bürglen L, Reboullet S et al. (1995) Identification and characterization of a spinal muscular atrophy-determining gene. Cell 80: 155–165.

Lefebvre S, Burlet P, Liu Q et al. (1997) Correlation between severity and SMN protein level in spinal muscular atrophy. Nature Genet 16: 265–269.

Lefebvre S, Bürglen L, Munnich A, Melki J (1998) The role of the SMN gene in proximal spinal muscular atrophy. Hum Mol Genet 7: 1531–1536.

Liskay RM, Letsou A, Stachelek J (1987) Homology requirement for efficient gene conversion between duplicated chromosomal sequences in mammalian cells. Genetics 115: 161–167.

Liu Q, Dreyfuss G (1996) A novel nuclear structure containing the survival of motor neurons protein. EMBO J 15: 3555–3565.

Liu Q, Fischer U, Wang F, Dreyfuss G (1997) The spinal muscular atrophy gene product, SMN, and its associated protein SIP1 are in a complex with spliceosomal snRNP proteins. Cell 90: 1013–1021.

Lorson CL, Androphy EJ (1998) The domain encoded by exon 2 of the survival motor neuron protein mediates nucleic acid binding. Hum Mol Genet 7: 1269–1275.

Lorson CL, Strasswimmer J, Yao J et al. (1998) SMN oligomerization defect correlates with spinal muscular atrophy severity. Nature Genet 19: 63–66.

Mattaj IW (1998) Ribonucleoprotein assembly: clues from spinal muscular atrophy. Curr Biol 8: R93–R95.

McAndrew PE, Parsons DW, Simard LR et al. (1997) Identification of proximal spinal muscular atrophy carriers and patients by analysis of SMN1 and SMN2 gene copy number. Am J Hum Genet 60: 1411–1422.

Melki J, Lefebvre S, Burglen L et al. (1994) De novo and inherited deletions of the 5q13 region in spinal muscular atrophies. Science 264(5164): 1474–1477.

Monani UR, Sendtner M, Coovert DD (2000) The Human Centromeric survival motor neuron gene (SMN2) rescues embryonic lethality in Smn/mice and results in a mouse with Spinal muscular atrophy. Human Molecular Genetics 9:333–339.

Moosa A, Dubowitz V (1973) Spinal muscular atrophy in childhood. Arch Dis Child 48: 386–388.

Munsat TL (1991) International SMA collaboration. Neuromusc Disord 1: 81.

Parsons DW, McAndrew PE, Iannaccone ST, Mendell JR, Burghes AH, Prior TW (1998a) Intragenic telSMN mutations: frequency, distribution, evidence of a founder effect, and modification of the spinal muscular atrophy phenotype by cenSMN copy number. Am J Hum Genet 63: 1712–1723.

Parsons DW, McAndrew PE, Allinson PS, Parker WD, Burghes AHM, Prior TW (1998b) Diagnosis of spinal muscular atrophy in an SMN non-deletion patient using a quantitative PCR screen and mutation analysis. J Med Genet 35: 674–676.

Pearn J (1980) Classification of spinal muscular atrophies. Lancet 1: 919–922.

Pellizzoni L, Kataoka N, Charroux B, Dreyfuss G (1998) A novel function for SMN, the spinal muscular atrophy disease gene product, in pre-mRNA splicing. Cell 95: 615–624.

Rodrigues NR, Owen N, Talbot K et al. (1996) Gene deletions in spinal muscular atrophy. J Med Genet 33: 93–96.

Roy N, Mahadevan MS, McLean M et al. (1995) The gene for neuronal apoptosis inhibitory protein is partially deleted in individuals with spinal muscular atrophy. Cell 80: 167–178.

Rudnick-Schöneborn S, Lutzenrath S, Borkowska J, Karwanska A, Hausmanowa-Petrusewicz I, Zerres K (1998) Analysis of creatine kinase activity in 504 patients with proximal spinal muscular atrophy types I-III from the point of view of progression and severity. Eur Neurol 39: 154–162.

Russman BS, Iannaccone ST, Buncher CR et al. (1992) Spinal muscular atrophy: new thoughts on the pathogenesis and classification schema. J Child Neurol 7: 347–353.

Russman BS, Buncher CR, Samaha F, Iannaccone ST, DCN/SMA Group (1996) Function changes in spinal muscular atrophy II and III. Neurology 47: 973–976.

Scharf JM, Endrizzi MG, Wetter A et al. (1998) Identification of a candidate modifying gene for spinal muscular atrophy by comparitive genomics. Nature Genet 20: 83–86.

Schrank B, Götz R, Gunnersen JM et al. (1997) Inactivation of the survival motor neuron gene, a candidate gene for human spinal muscular atrophy, leads to massive cell death in early mouse embryos. Proc Natl Acad Sci USA 94: 9920–9925.

Simard LR, Rochette C, Semionov A, Morgan K, Vanasse M (1997) SMN(T) and NAIP mutations in Canadian families with spinal muscular atrophy (SMA): genotype/phenotype correlations with disease severity. Am J Hum Genet 72: 51–58.

Talbot K, Ponting CP, Theodosiou AM et al. (1997) Missense mutation clustering in the survival motor neuron gene: a role for a conserved tyrosine and glycine rich region of the protein in RNA metabolism? Hum Mol Genet 6: 497–500.

Taylor JE, Thomas NH, Lewis CM et al. (1998) Correlation of SMNt and SMNc gene copy number with age of onset and survival in spinal muscular atrophy. Eur J Hum Genet 6: 467–474.

Thomas NH, Dubowitz V (1994) The natural history of type I (severe) spinal muscular atrophy. Neuromus Disord 4: 497–502.

Thompson TG, DiDonato CJ, Simard LR et al. (1995) A novel cDNA detects homozygous microdeletions in greater than 50% of type I spinal muscular atrophy patients. Nature Genet 9: 56–62.

Towfighi J, Young RSK, Ward RM (1985) Is Werdnig–Hoffmann disease a pure lower motor neuron disorder? Acta Neuropathol (Berl) 65: 270–280.

van der Steege G, Grootscholten PM, van der Vlies P et al. (1995) PCR-based DNA test to confirm clinical diagnosis of autosomal recessive spinal muscular atrophy. Lancet 345: 985–986.

Velasco E, Valero C, Valero A, Moreno F, Hernandezchico C (1996) Molecular analysis of the SMN and NAIP genes in Spanish spinal muscular atrophy (SMA) families and correlation between number of copies of cBCD541 and SMA phenotype. Hum Mol Genet 5: 257–263.

Wang CH, Carter TA, Ross BM et al. (1996) Characterization of survival motor neuron (SMN^T) gene deletions in asymptomatic carriers of spinal muscular atrophy. Hum Mol Genet 5: 359–365.

Wang CH, Carter TA, Das K et al. (1997) Extensive DNA deletion associated with severe disease alleles on spinal muscular atrophy homologues. Ann Neurol 42: 41–49.

Watnick TJ, Gandolph MA, Weber H, Neumann HPH, Germino GG (1998) Gene conversion is a likely cause of mutation in PKD1. Hum Mol Genet 7: 1239–1243.

Werdnig G (1891) Zwei fruhinfantile hereditare falle von progressiver muskelatrophie unter dem bilde der dystrophie, aber auf neurotischer grundlage. Arch Psych Nervenkrank 22: 437–480.

Wirth B, Schmidt T, Hahnen E et al. (1997) De novo arrangements found in 2% of index patients with spinal muscular atrophy: mutational mechanisms, parental origin, mutation rate, and implications for genetic counseling. An J Hum Genet 61(5): 1102–1111.

Xu DG, Crocker SJ, Doucet J-P et al. (1997a) Elevation of neuronal expression of NAIP reduces ischemic damage in the hippocampus. Nature Med 3: 997–1003.

Xu DG, Korneluk RG, Tamai K et al. (1997b) Distribution of NAIP-like immunoreactivity in the rat central nervous system. J Comp Neurol 381: 1–13.

Zerres K, Rudnik-Schöneborn S, Forkert R, Wirth B (1995) Genetic basis of adult-onset spinal muscular atrophy. Lancet 346: 1162.

Zerres K, Wirth B, Rudnik-Schöneborn S (1997) Spinal muscular atrophy – clinical and genetic correlations. Neuromusc Disord 7: 202–207.

CHAPTER 6

Pharmacotherapy of ALS and its scientific basis

Jacques Hugon, Albert Ludolph, and Ralph W. Kuncl

Introduction

The pathophysiology of amyotrophic lateral sclerosis (ALS) is still mostly unknown but recent years have brought new insights into the molecular and cellular mechanisms leading to selective motor neuron death. The reason why upper and lower motor neurons are specifically involved in ALS still remains a mystery and represents a major hurdle to establish an ideal experimental model of this disease. Models are necessary to carry out preclinical studies with new drugs or biological tools (Louvel et al., 1997). Different experimental models have distinct advantages and limitations (Ludolph, 1996) (Table 6.1). It should be emphasized that transgenic mice carrying a human mutation of the SOD1 gene observed in familial ALS represent a major advance. These mice display neuropathological features reminiscent of the human spinal cord pathology detected in ALS (Gurney et al., 1994). This model is likely to be used more extensively in the future for drug screening (Wong et al., 1995) or transgenic therapy, as recently published (Gurney et al., 1996; Kostic et al., 1997). Other in vitro models have certain pathophysiologic value for sporadic ALS, as they focus for example on spinal cord lesions induced by glutamate (Rothstein and Kuncl, 1995) or neuronal lesions produced by the cerebrospinal fluid (CSF) of ALS patients (Couratier et al., 1993). Such models help bring drugs to clinical trials. In this chapter we will review the literature concerning the recent clinical trials carried out in ALS patients with anti-excitotoxic or related neuroprotective drugs and with neurotrophic agents, which are the major current trends in pharmacotherapy.

Anti-excitotoxic drugs
Rationale

The causes of ALS are still not elucidated, but during the last 10 years a growing body of evidence has suggested that glutamate toxicity (or excitotoxicity)

Table 6.1 Models of motor neuron disease

Models (ref)	Species	Pathological lesions
Axotomy (Sendtner et al., 1990)	Newborn rat or chick	Motor neuron apoptosis
Toxic models		
• Intrathecal kainate toxicity (Hugon et al., 1989)	Rat	Lower motor neuron degeneration
• BOAA (Spencer et al., 1986)	Monkey	Corticospinal tract deficits
• BMAA (Spencer et al., 1987)	Monkey	Upper and lower motor neuron lesion
• IDPN (Chou and Harman, 1964)	Rat	Neurofilament accumulations in axons
Genetic models		
• Wobbler (Mitsumoto and Pioro, 1995)	Mouse	Vacuolar degeneration of motor neurons
• pmn (Schmalbruch et al., 1991)	Mouse	Possible motor neuropathy
• Mnd (Messer and Flaherty, 1986)	Mouse	Multisystem neuronal degeneration
• Hereditary canine spinal muscular atrophy (Cork et al., 1979)	Dog	Axonal pathology of lower motor neurons
Transgenic models		
• SOD1 mutation (Gurney et al., 1994)	Mouse	Vacuolar degeneration of motor neurons
• Neurofilament mutation (Côte et al., 1993)	Mouse	Neurofilamentous swellings in motor neurons and axons
Cellular models		
• Organotypic spinal cord cultures (Rothstein and Kuncl, 1995)	Rat	Slow glutamate-mediated motor neuron vacuolar degeneration
• Primary neuronal cultures (Couratier et al., 1993)	Rat	ALS CSF toxicity
Immunological models (Appel et al., 1995)	Guinea pig	Upper and lower motor neuron lesions

could play a role in the origin of neuropathological lesions observed in patients. Glutamate is one of the major excitatory neurotransmitters in the brain but also a potent neurotoxin. Glutamate acts on three types of postsynaptic receptors: NMDA, AMPA/kainate and metabotropic receptors. Clinical and experimental findings in a remote and largely unknown disease, lathyrism, has led to the association between excitatory amino acids and motor disorders of the central nervous system (Ludolph et al., 1987). Lathyrism is clinically characterized by the sudden or progressive onset of spastic paraplegia in subjects eating *Lathyrus sativus*. The motor tract disorder is reproduced experimentally in monkeys fed for several months either with *Lathyrus sativus* or the excitatory neurotoxin β-oxalylamino-L-alanine, which it contains (Spencer et al., 1986; Hugon et al., 1988). Similarly, Guam ALS was associated with another excitotoxin, β-methylamino-L-alanine, although a causal link is not proven (Spencer et al., 1987). Abnormal glutamate metabolism was described more than a decade ago in patients with ALS (Plaitakis and Caroscio, 1987; Hugon et al., 1989). Elevated CSF levels of glutamate and aspartate in ALS, first reported by the laboratory of Kuncl and colleagues (Rothstein et al., 1990), were ultimately attributed to defective glutamate uptake in the motor cortex and spinal cord (Rothstein et al., 1992) due to decreased expression of the glial glutamate transporter GLT1 (Rothstein et al., 1995). The excitotoxic activity of CSF was mediated by AMPA/kainate glutamate receptors; this was detectable in ALS patients but not in patients with other neurodegenerative disorders or in control patients without chronic neurological diseases (Couratier et al., 1993). All these findings led several clinical groups during recent years to undertake clinical trials in ALS patients using anti-excitotoxic chemicals known to interfere with glutamatergic transmission.

Fast or slow excitotoxicity are now implicated in the pathophysiology of a large variety of neurological disorders, including stroke, epilepsy, Huntington's disease, Alzheimer's disease, Parkinson's disease and ALS (Choi, 1988). The slow degeneration of postsynaptic neurons is linked to the chronic over activation of glutamate receptors in relation to enhanced release or decreased reuptake of glutamate in the synaptic cleft. Neurons in acute pathological conditions, such as chemical hypoxia, may also become more sensitive to normal extracellular concentrations of glutamate. The goal of anti-excitotoxic drug use is to protect neurons from the deleterious effects of glutamate release in the synapse (Zorumski and Olney, 1993).

Dextromethorphan

Dextromethorphan, commonly used as an antitussive, is an NMDA antagonist that reduces neuronal degeneration in an experimental model of cerebral ischemia (Steinberg, 1991) and also possesses antiepileptic properties (Wong et al., 1987). Several studies, all negative, were carried out using dextromethorphan in ALS patients. Askmark et al. (1993) enrolled 14 ALS patients in a double-blind cross-over clinical trial. Patients received 150 mg dextromethorphan daily or placebo for 12 weeks, with a wash-out period of 4 weeks between treatments. Then, all patients received 100 mg dextromethorphan daily for up to 6 months in an open trial. Outcome was evaluated with the aid of the Norris scale and bulbar and spinal scores. Neurophysiological parameters were also assessed, such as the amplitude and area of the compound action muscle potential of the abductor digiti minimi muscle. No differences were observed between dextromethorphan or placebo-treated groups based on clinical and neurophysiological evaluations. Blin et al. (1996) studied dextromethorphan (1.5 mg/kg) for a 1-year period. This double-blind placebo-controlled study enrolling 49 patients did not detect any differences in the rate of clinical deterioration between the groups treated with dextromethorphan or placebo, as assessed by the Norris scale. The authors suggested that higher doses or other potent NMDA receptor antagonists should be used. Gredal et al. (1997) reported using dextromethorphan at the dose of 150 mg per day in a double-blind placebo-controlled study of 45 ALS patients. Patients were followed for 1 year using survival rate, decline in pulmonary function, and functional disability. Except for a significantly less pronounced rate of decline in the disability scores for the lower extremities in the dextromethorphan group, no differences were noted between the two groups, including the survival rate.

Lamotrigine

The drug lamotrigine (3,5-diamino-6-(2,3 dichlorophenyl)-1,2,4-triazine) acts on voltage sensitive sodium channels and reduces the release of glutamate from presynaptic terminals (Brodie, 1992). Lamotrigine is used as an antiepileptic drug in neurological practice. In 1993, Eisen et al. reported the results of a double-blind placebo-controlled study in ALS patients using lamotrigine at the oral daily dose of 100 mg (Eisen et al., 1993). A total of 67 patients were enrolled for a 1.5-year period. No significant differences were noted between the two groups in survival rate, clinical scores, and cortical threshold or motor evoked potential/compound action muscle potential ratios after cortical magnetic stimulation. The authors pointed out that an effect on fasciculations was observed in the lamotrigine group. The dose of lamotrigine used (100 mg per day) was rather moderate but, according to the authors, difficult to increase because of undesirable side effects.

Gabapentin

Gabapentin is an anticonvulsant drug, but the exact mechanisms interfering with glutamatergic neurotransmission are still not fully elucidated. Gabapentin may reduce releasable glutamate and thus decrease glutamate excitotoxicity. This drug has a modest neuroprotective effect on tissue cultures against glutamate toxicity (Rothstein and Kuncl, 1995) and prolongs survival in the familial ALS model of *SOD1* transgenic mice (Gurney et al., 1996). In an initial trial, Miller et al. (1996b) enrolled 152 ALS patients (all with definite or probable ALS by El Escorial criteria) in a randomized placebo-controlled double-blind study for 6 months. Outcome measures were the average maximum voluntary isometric strength from eight arm muscles standardized against a reference population (arm megascore) and the forced vital capacity. The authors observed a statistically nonsignificant trend toward a slower decline of muscle strength in patients treated with gabapentin compared to placebo. No difference was noted in the forced vital capacity. The only significant side effects in the gabapentin group were lightheadedness, fatigue, and drowsiness. The authors concluded that the study demonstrated a trend toward slowing the decline of arm strength in patients taking gabapentin and that the result supported the need for further study of this drug in ALS. That follow-up multicenter trial of 204 patients tested the efficacy of 3600 mg gabapentin per day for 9 months in a definitive study (Miller et al., 2001), but unfortunately it failed to demonstrate the anticipated clinical benefit. There was no significant slowing of the decline in muscle strength, change in pulmonary function, nor change in symptoms.

Topiramate, a similar well tolerated anticonvulsant with potential antiglutamate mechanisms, is being tried in a large multicenter study of some 300 patients with ALS.

Branched chain amino acids

Several studies were undertaken in past years to analyze the effects of branched chain amino acids in ALS. The rationale was based on the finding that a partial deficiency of glutamate dehydrogenase can occur in patients with some neurodegenerative diseases and branched chain amino acids can activate the enzyme. Glutamate dehydrogenase activity was found decreased in a subset of ALS patients (Hugon et al., 1988). In 1988, Plaitakis et al. reported an improvement in ALS patients treated daily with 12 g L-leucine, 8 g L-isoleucine, and 6.4 g L-valine orally (Plaitakis et al., 1988). Unfortunately, later studies did not confirm these results and an apparent increased mortality of ALS patients in an Italian study led to an early cessation of this therapeutic trial (Testa et al., 1989).

L-Threonine

Nearly two decades ago, a report showed that L-threonine administration enhanced glycine levels in the 'rat central nervous system (Maher and Wurtman, 1980). Since glycine is an inhibitory neurotransmitter in the human spinal cord, L-threonine was given to patients with familial spastic paraparesis (Nader et al., 1987). This amino acid produced an increased concentration of glycine in the CSF and reduced spasticity in treated patients. Based on these findings, L-threonine was proposed to antagonize excitatory neurotransmission in ALS. Several studies were carried out with ALS patients using oral doses of L-threonine up to 6 g per day (Patten et al., 1988; Blin et al., 1992; Hugon et al., 1992). Clinical scores were assessed up to 12 months, and no differences were noted between placebo and L-threonine groups. At the onset of treatment patients seemed to 'feel better' but L-threonine did not modify the evolution of the disease.

Riluzole

Riluzole is a neuroprotective chemical that reduces glutamatergic transmission in the central nervous system. This drug blocks the voltage-dependent sodium channel. Riluzole attenuates glutamate release from brain slices, from corticostriatal neurons *in vivo*, and from cultured neuronal cells. A recent review has underlined the multiple potential neuroprotective properties of riluzole (Doble, 1996). The rationale for using it in ALS was reinforced by the positive effects of this drug in three preclinical models. Riluzole prevents neuronal degeneration of cultured cells induced by the CSF from ALS patients (Couratier et al., 1994). Another study reported that this drug is a potent neuroprotectant in a model of chronic glutamate-mediated motor neuron toxicity using organotypic spinal cord cultures (Rothstein and Kuncl, 1995). Finally, in a model of familial ALS using *SOD1* transgenic mice, recent work revealed that riluzole prolongs survival of transgenic mice but does not delay the onset of the disease (Gurney et al., 1996).

Two recent clinical trials have shown that riluzole prolongs survival in ALS patients. The first clinical trial was carried out in 1994 and enrolled 155 ALS patients (Bensimon et al., 1994). In this prospective double-blind placebo-controlled study each patient received 100 mg riluzole or placebo for a period of at least 12 months. The primary endpoints were survival and the rate of changes in clinical scores. At the end of the 12-month period, 58% of patients were still alive in the placebo group (45/78) and 74% of patients were alive in the riluzole group (57/77). The treatment effect appeared more pronounced in patients with a bulbar-onset disease than in patients with limb-onset disease. Asthenia, stiffness and increased aminotransferase levels in the blood were among the notable side effects. The rate of muscle deterioration was positively modified by riluzole. In the second, confirmatory dose-ranging trial using riluzole, 959 outpatients were included (Lacomblez et al., 1996). The design of the study was similar to the first trial. Patients received 50, 100, 200 mg riluzole or placebo for up to 18 months. The results confirm that riluzole demonstrates a dose-dependent positive effect on survival. No bulbar effect was seen in this study. At the dose of 100 mg per day, and after adjustment for significant prognostic factors, the risk of death or tracheostomy was decreased by 35% over an 18-month period in patients treated with riluzole compared to placebo. Riluzole was approved in the USA and Europe, and to date riluzole is still the only approved drug to modify the course of ALS.

Other potentially neuroprotective drugs acting on mitochondria, oxidative stress, calcium, or apoptosis

Several neuroprotective drugs already available on the market were tested recently in ALS patients. The rationale for using these drugs was based on the findings that free radicals could be involved in the pathophysiology of a subset of familial ALS with *SOD1* mutations and that intracellular calcium concentrations can play a role in some aspects of neuronal degeneration linked to excitotoxicity or free radical toxicity. Mitochondria are central to the processes of free radical generation and calcium homeostasis (see related discussion in Chapter 3); mitochondria are themselves particularly vulnerable to oxidative stress. Transgenic mice carrying the G93A human *SOD1* mutation exhibit altered electron transport and early mitochondrial swelling and vacuolization; expression of the mutant enzyme *in vitro* results in loss of mitochondrial membrane potential and elevated cytoplasmic concentrations of calcium.

N-Acetylcysteine

N-Acetylcysteine is a free radical scavenger and was used at the dose of 50 mg/kg in a double-blind placebo-controlled study enrolling 111 patients. Clinical scores, pulmonary function, and survival were used for the assessment of evolution during 12 months. N-Acetylcysteine did not induce a significant increase in survival or slowing of the disease (Louwerse et al., 1995).

Creatine

If mitochondrial dysfunction leads to motor neuron energy depletion in ALS, then buffering intracellular energy levels could exert a neuroprotective influence. Creatine monohydrate administration provides the carrier for high energy phosphates as creatine phosphate, and together with creatine kinase they constitute an energy buffering and transport system connecting the sites of energy production in mitochondria and sites of energy consumption throughout the cell. Creatine stabilizes the mitochondrial creatine kinase and inhibits opening of the mitochondrial transition pore. In G93A transgenic ALS mice, oral administration of creatine extended survival minimally, ameliorated the loss of motor neurons slightly, attenuated the increases in markers of oxidative damage, and produced a small dose-dependent improvement in motor performance (Klivenyi et al., 1999). It is important to note that, although these effects were small, they were internally consistent. Brief clinical trials in patients with a variety of muscular dystrophies demonstrated that saturating doses of creatine for brief periods significantly increased muscle power (Walter et al., 2000); again, the effect was small, of the order of 4%, which is an amount statistically significant but not clinically perceptible by individual patients or their physicians. On the strength of this preclinical rationale, many patients with ALS are taking creatine supplementation, in the absence of a proper clinical trial (Tarnopolsky and Beal, 2001).

Coenzyme Q_{10}

This is an essential factor of the electron transport chain and a potent free radical scavenger in mitochondrial membranes. It was shown to prolong lifespan slightly in the transgenic mouse model of ALS (Matthews et al., 1998). It is available in health food stores and, like vitamin E and C and other weak 'natural' antioxidants, has not been tested in human double-blind placebo-controlled studies of ALS. As with creatine (above), the value of novel bioenergetic transfer therapies is unknown in human ALS but widely touted in a variety of neurodegenerative diseases (Tarnopolsky and Beal, 2001).

Calcium channel antagonists

Two studies were published in 1996 by Miller et al. using verapamil or nimodipine (Miller et al., 1996d,e). No significant differences were noted concerning pulmonary function and limb strength between the control groups and groups receiving verapamil or nimodipine.

Selegiline

Selegiline is a neuroprotective drug of potential interest in Parkinson's disease (Langston, 1990). Three studies were undertaken using selegiline in ALS patients (Jossan et al., 1994; Mazzini et al., 1994; Lange et al., 1998). Unfortunately, in double-blind placebo-controlled studies, selegiline does not appear to modify the evolution of ALS.

Anti-apoptosis drugs

Because programmed cell death could also be involved in degenerative diseases of the nervous system (Leist and Nicotera, 1998), anti-apoptotic drugs are also proposed. Although the role of apoptosis in sporadic ALS (Martin, 1999, 2000) is itself rather controversial, an experimental caspase inhibitor drug which might be expected to reduce apoptosis, zVAD-fmk, has indeed substantially delayed symptom onset and prolonged survival in the transgenic ALS mouse (Li et al., 2000). On this and other rationales, an exploratory clinical trial of minocycline has begun, as minocycline inhibits the activity of inducible nitric oxide synthase and caspase enzymes (which play roles in apoptosis). This is a simplistic approach, as the promoting or negating direction of the nuanced roles of caspases and transcription factors within the complex process of programmed cell death are dependent on the model studied.

Summary

Until now, only one anti-excitotoxic drug, riluzole, has shown some mild efficacy in modifying the course of human ALS. If deleterious consequences of AMPA/kainate receptor activation play a role in the pathogenesis of ALS, it will be very useful to test new nonNMDA antagonists acting on these receptors in ALS patients, if such drugs can be found that do not have severely limiting toxicity. Future directions may also include the modification of metabotropic receptor activities. So far, the anti-oxidant, anti-calcium, anti-apoptosis, and bioenergetic transfer strategies have not matured in clinical trials.

Other future trends are discussed in detail in Chapter 9. A useful way to keep abreast of modern clinical trial strategies and availability is to consult the World Federation of Neurology's ALS website at *www.wfnals.org*, which includes the Amyotrophic Lateral Sclerosis Association's 'Drug Development Update' database.

Neurotrophic strategies
Rationale

In the early 1990s, experimental evidence in inherited mouse models of diseases selectively affecting the motor system, such as the *wobbler* and *pmn* mice, supported the concept that growth factors could play a role in future therapeutic approaches to human motor neuron diseases (Sendtner et al., 1992; Mitsumoto et al., 1994; Ikeda et al., 1995; Sagot et al., 1995). By using recombinant protein, treatment strategies were quickly evaluated in large human trials which were, however, unsuccessful if the high expectations are considered. Therefore enthusiasm is currently tempered and replaced by scepticism; however, final conclusions can only be drawn when elements that may have prevented immediate success, such as pharmacokinetics, dosage, bioavailability, target cells, systemic toxic effects, and neurotoxicity, are carefully explored for the growing number of clinically relevant growth factors (Hefti, 1997). Recent evidence indicates that the question whether growth factors can be successfully delivered to the central nervous system by appropriate viral vectors needs to be addressed (see Chapter 9). Side effects and risks of therapeutic approaches with growth factors will have to be carefully defined, and their differential effects on energy-depleted cells and resulting necrotic and apoptotic cell death need to be differentiated (Koh et al., 1995). Therefore, neurotrophic strategies are currently not a factor in the standard pharmacotherapy of ALS, but they remain promising therapeutic agents and clearly merit further consideration. Mitsumoto and Tsuzaka (1999a,b) have reviewed the subject in detail.

CNTF

Ciliary derived neurotrophic factor (CNTF) was the first growth factor speculated to be relevant for ALS therapy, when it was shown to prevent degeneration of motor neurons in the rat after axotomy (Sendtner et al., 1990). Experiments in the *pmn* mouse model demonstrated that CNTF slowed down degeneration of the motor system (Sendtner et al., 1992). In combination with brain-derived neurotrophic factor (BDNF) it seemed to arrest the course of the disease in the *wobbler* mutant. A phase I–II clinical trial was apparently promising, and acceptable side effects in humans were observed. However, a large phase II–III trial (subcutaneous application of either 30 or 15 µg/kg rhCNTF thrice weekly) clearly failed to show efficacy (ALS CNTF Treatment Study Group, 1996), and a second one had to be discontinued because of intolerable side effects (Miller et al., 1996a). In the completed study, measurement of isometric muscle strength as a primary endpoint showed that CNTF-treated patients developed a significant deterioration of muscle strength compared with controls in the early phases of the study, and in later stages no differences from controls were detected. Also, mortality, pulmonary function, and patients' functional abilities were not influenced by CNTF (ALS CNTF Treatment Study Group, 1996). Side effects such as anorexia, nausea, weight loss, asthenia, increased salivation, aphthous stomatitis, and cough appeared dose-related and thus limited treatment in a number of patients, in particular in early phases of the disease (ALS CNTF Treatment Study Group, 1996). Injection site reactions were seen. At the highest doses, the death rate appeared to increase, but this was not statistically significant. In the second four-armed study, 0.5, 2, or 5 µg/kg/day CNTF or placebo was administered subcutaneously to 570 patients for 6 months (Miller et al., 1996a). Efficacy could not be detected at any of the dosages studied, and the profile of adverse effects was similar to that in the first study. However, in the highest dose group, adverse events and premature withdrawals were seen more frequently and the death rate was statistically significantly increased when compared with controls. Increased death rate was also observed in the 1-month follow-up period.

The lack of efficacy of CNTF in clinical trials has been attributed to several factors. The protein has a short half life in the circulation and may be unable to cross the blood–brain barrier at the dosages used (Dittrich et al., 1994). It remains possible that CNTF is taken up at the neuromuscular junction and transported retrogradely to the perikaryon (Curtis et al., 1993). Furthermore, antibodies develop during CNTF treatment. In the first study (ALS CNTF Treatment Study Group, 1996), more than 75% of the patients remaining in the study during the full 9-month period developed circulating antibodies to rhCNTF, which are of unknown significance for the effects and side effects observed. It is noteworthy that the time of appearance of antibodies coincided with the reduction of frequency and severity of early side effects, in particular the weight loss and consistent reduction of muscle strength (ALS CNTF Treatment Study Group, 1996, Miller et al., 1996a).

Further studies of CNTF side effects revealed that the aphthous stomatitis was associated with a recurrence of HSV-1 infections, which were apparently more severe than previous episodes experienced by individual patients (Miller et al.,

1996b). In a single patient, aseptic meningitis was seen during CNTF treatment, but HSV-1 was neither isolated nor identified (Miller et al., 1996a).

To summarize, positive effects of CNTF in traditional experimental models of motor neuron diseases did not find their counterpart in patients suffering from ALS. Studies of the effects of CNTF on transgenic mice carrying human Cu/Zn SOD mutations have apparently not been done. It is a second lesson from these first clinical applications that significant side effects of the drug at the dosage used – including increased death rates—need to be considered if CNTF is to be applied with novel forms of administration such as intrathecal delivery or with the aid of adenoviral vectors in the future.

BDNF

BDNF is a target-derived protein which reportedly retards motor dysfunction in *wobbler* mouse motor neuron disease, an established hereditary model of premature motor neuron loss (Ikeda et al., 1995). If these mice are cotreated with CNTF and BDNF, disease progression seems to arrest for one month (Mitsumoto et al., 1994). However, knock-out mice lacking BDNF do not develop motor deficits but rather develop deficits of vestibular and sensory neuronal populations (Conover et al., 1995).

Recombinant brain-derived neurotrophic factor (rhBDNF) has been applied subcutaneously to ALS patients in three large studies. Since deterioration of forced vital capacity could be slowed down by multiple dose subcutaneous application in a phase II study during a follow-up period of 6 months, a second study was initiated (Bernstein et al., 1997). Disappointingly, subcutaneous daily application of 25 or 100 µg/kg body weight rhBDNF did not result in any benefit for the primary endpoints of survival and respiratory function (Bernstein et al., 1997; Cedarbaum et al., 1998). One possible explanation was insufficient permeability of the blood–brain barrier for this and other growth factors (Poduslo and Curran, 1996), although evidence exists for retrograde and anterograde transport of BDNF in the peripheral and central nervous system (Altar et al., 1997). A post-hoc subgroup analysis of the trial appeared to show efficacy in those high-dose patients who experienced gastrointestinal side effects, suggesting a dose/level effect. On that basis, a third study was designed to test high dose escalation to the limits of side effects. At the same time, an intrathecal study was designed. After intrathecal administration BDNF accumulates in spinal motor neurons, obviating the limitations of dose, distribution, and retrograde transport associated with systemic administration (Dittrich et al., 1996). Early experience indicated that the spectrum of side effects was apparently different from that seen after subcutaneous application and included reversible paresthesias and sleep disturbances (Ochs et al., 1998). Intrathecal delivery clearly permits the compound to reach the central nervous system, in particular anterior horn cells (Ochs et al., 1998). Both the high dose subcutaneous and the intrathecal studies were discontinued early by the respective independent monitoring boards when it became clear that neither study's primary endpoints of survival or ventilator use could reach statistical significance for efficacy (Amgen-Regeneron Partners press release, January 25, 2001). Thus, BDNF – like CNTF – has not yet fulfilled initial expectations.

IGF-1

Insulin-like growth factor 1 (IGF-1) is a factor with pluripotent effects on the entire motor unit, as it has trophic actions on the motor neuron, motor nerve, neuromuscular junction, and muscle (Vaught et al., 1996). IGF-1 increases embryonic motor neuron survival in culture and reduces naturally occurring embryonic motor neuron death *in vivo* (Neff et al., 1993). IGF-1 is known to promote motor neuron survival *in vivo*, to increase ChAT activity in embryonic rat spinal cord cultures, and to protect embryonic motor neurons from differentation or axotomy-induced death (Neff et al., 1993). These preclinical models have limited inference for late adult degenerative diseases. However, even in more mature motor neurons in organotypic spinal cord cultures, IGF-1 increases motor neuron ChAT activity (Corse et al., 1999). In such cultures, excess glutamate levels induced by long-term inhibition of glutamate transport cause a slow death of motor neurons (Rothstein et al., 1993). In this model of mature motor neuron degeneration, IGF-1 is potently neuroprotective (Corse et al., 1999). By comparison, in the same model, CNTF, BDNF, and neurotrophin-3 (NT-3) failed, whereas glial-derived neurotrophic factor (GDNF), its analog neurturin, and pigment epithelium-derived factor (PEDF) succeeded (Bilak et al., 1999a, b; Corse et al., 1999).

Recombinant human (rh) IGF-1 has been studied in humans in two large multicenter placebo-controlled, double-blind, randomized clinical trials. In the North American study, three parallel groups received placebo, 50 or 100 µg/kg rhIGF-1 by daily subcutaneous injection (Lange, 1996; Lai et al., 1997). In the European trial only the larger dosage was used (Borasio et al., 1998). The therapeutic effect of the drug on the Appel scale – a widely accepted functional scale – was the primary outcome measure in each trial. In the North American trial, slowing of functional decline was convincingly demonstrated and furthermore was dose responsive. The European trial revealed a trend in the same direction which did not reach statistical significance at the $P < 0.05$ level. However, a pooled analysis of patients having received 0.1 mg/kg/day in both trials showed an unequivocal beneficial effect on muscle strength and bulbar and upper extremity muscle function during disease progression (Leigh et al., 1997). Effects were more pronounced in patients with rapidly progressive disease (Leigh et al., 1997). In prospective analyses, no effect on survival could be shown in either study (Borasio et al., 1998; Lange, 1996; Lai et al., 1997). Although the North American trial was not designed to measure survival as a primary outcome, analysis of extended follow-up data using a stratified logrank analysis, taking into account age and forced vital capacity as prognostic indicators, suggested a possible survival benefit of the drug. The usual caveats apply to this post-hoc analysis.

Intravenous injection of IGF-1 is associated with serious side effects on the cardiovascular system, but subcutaneous injections of up to 120 µg/kg body weight are apparently safe (Le Roith, 1997). Hypoglycemia is a consistent significant side effect of rhIGF-1, which can be avoided by careful monitoring of blood glucose levels and timing of injections in relation to meals (Le Roith, 1997). In the IGF-1 trials the dosages employed were reportedly tolerable, and less than 4% of patients had to discontinue treatment. If IGF-1 is to be employed in more chronic diseases, potential long-term side effects such as acromegaly, tissue hypertrophy, or even tumor cell proliferation need to be addressed (Le Roith, 1997, Chan et al., 1998). The wide range of biological effects of rhIGF-1, in particular its anabolic effects, raises the question of whether the therapeutic benefit that was clearly detected in the pooled analysis of both IGF-1 studies was related to an effect on the motor neuron, its axons, skeletal muscle, or other organs.

In summary, IGF-1 seems to be the first drug for ALS which has been shown to affect strength and functional outcome (see Chapter 8); however, whether this effect is due to a neuroprotective effect on motor neurons is not yet known. *In vitro* modeling suggests it is (Corse et al., 1999). A third study of IGF-1 alone or in combination with riluzole may be necessary to prove a potential effect of the drug on survival and gain its approval.

GDNF

GDNF, initially identified as a potent trophic factor for ventral midbrain dopaminergic neurons (Lin et al., 1993), is now recognized to be the most potent survival factor for motor neurons. It is approximately two orders of magnitude more potent than the neurotrophins in promoting survival of motor neurons in chick embryos *in vitro*, in neonatal rats following axotomy, and in postnatal organotypic spinal cord undergoing slow excitotoxic degeneration (Zurn et al., 1994; Oppenheim et al., 1995; Yan et al., 1995; Milbrandt et al., 1998; Corse et al., 1999). GDNF also potently evokes neurite outgrowth from ventral spinal motor neurons (Bilak et al., 1999b). It was modestly effective in the *wobbler* mouse model (Mitsumoto and Tsuzaka, 1999). So far, intrathecal GDNF has only been explored in a small group of patients with ALS, and unpublished results were said to be uninformative (Mitsumoto and Tsuzaka, 1999a, b). GDNF trials in ALS, though rational and based on a wealth of preclinical data, will probably not mature unless the more pressing ongoing clinical trials in Parkinson's disease and progressive supranuclear palsy are completed successfully.

Human growth hormone

In an early small study, the effect of recombinant human growth hormone on ALS was examined in 75 patients (Smith et al., 1993). Weekly administration of 0.3 mg/kg human growth hormone over 12–18 months did not show any benefit on the primary endpoint of survival or on established functional scales.

Other neurotrophic factors

Other neurotrophic factors are still in preclinical development. Neurturin, a homolog of GDNF, increases ChAT activity of normal postnatal motor neurons, induces neurite outgrowth in spinal cord, and potently protects postnatal motor neurons from chronic glutamate-mediated degeneration (Bilak et al., 1999b).

PEDF is an interesting novel growth factor. Originally derived from the pigmented epithelium of the retina, it has a much wider distribution in spinal motor neurons, skeletal muscle, and CSF (Bilak et al., 1999a), suggesting it may have autocrine and paracrine effects on motor neurons as well as being target derived. PEDF receptors occur on spinal motor neurons (Bilak et al., 2001b), and in the postnatal organotypic spinal cord model of slow motor neuron degeneration PEDF is highly neuroprotective (Bilak et al., 1999a). Efficacy can be accounted for entirely by a small 44-amino acid fragment of the molecule (Bilak et al., 1999c).

Non-peptide growth factor effectors: xaliproden

The prototype in this category is the molecule 1-(2-(napht-2-yl)ethyl)-4-(3-tri-fluoromethylphenyl)-1,2,5,6-tetrahydropyridine hydrochloride (xaliproden; previously named SR57746A). A neurotrophic effect of xaliproden has been shown in a number of animal models of neurodegenerative disorders (Fournier et al., 1993), including the ability of spinal cord explants to innervate muscle cells and the survival of *pmn* mice (Duong et al., 1998). Its action is presumably indirect, most probably caused by an increase of NGF and BDNF expression in various CNS regions (Fournier et al., 1998). The comparatively small compound is readily able to cross the blood–brain barrier. An initial phase II trial showed small but significant beneficial effects on the clinical course of ALS. This prompted two large simultaneous multicenter phase III trials which enrolled approximately 2000 patients who were treated for 18 months at 54 centers in Europe and North America. The drug was well tolerated but did not produce statistically significant benefits in the primary outcomes of survival (time to death, tracheostomy, or permanent assisted ventilation), or rate of progression of disease (unpublished data, Sanofi-Synthelabo Inc. press release, September 5, 2000, and www.fnals.org website).

Like xaliproden, the anxiolytic agent buspirone has a high affinity for serotonin receptors but may also mimic or stimulate the activity of endogenous neurotrophins such as NGF and BDNF. Tests in transgenic ALS mice and a small clinical trial are in progress.

Future directions

Although first attempts to introduce growth factors into clinical ALS therapy were largely unsuccessful, new forms of application might overcome difficulties in bioavailability and possibly alter toxicity. Trials of intrathecal application of factors such as BDNF, CNTF, and GDNF (Penn et al., 1997; Ochs et al., 1998) at least proved feasibility if not efficacy, so future intrathecal neurotrophic trials can be expected. However, the pattern of side effects can be expected to differ greatly from those seen after systemic application (Penn et al., 1997; Ochs et al., 1998). It was reported that the intramuscular injection of NT-3 adenoviral vector produced major therapeutic effects in the *pmn* mouse mutant. This strategy increased the lifespan of the mutant by 50% (40.0 to 61.3 days), a result which was further improved by coadministration of CNTF with NT-3 (66 days) (Haase et al., 1997). Results reported in a model of axotomized facial motor neurons are consistent with these findings (Gravel et al., 1997). However, a number of problems must be overcome before such a strategy for drug administration to the central nervous system will be of real practical value for growth factors and other compounds. The most important problems are the formation of viral antibodies, the development of antibodies to the respective growth factors, neurotoxicity, and the identification of specific target tissues (Sendtner, 1997).

Certain combinations of trophic factors may prove to be particularly synergistic. CNTF and NT-3 are additive in *pmn* mice (Haase et al., 1997), and CNTF and BDNF are additive in *wobbler* mice (Mitsumoto et al., 1994). GDNF and IGF-1 are additive in the organotypic spinal cord model of ALS (Bilak et al., 2001a), providing virtually complete motor neuron survival for months and lengthening the time window during which toxic degeneration of motor neurons can continue before treatment actually begins (Bilak and Kuncl, 2001). Although trophic factors no doubt work synergistically *in vivo*, and although combinations appear dramatically effective in *in vitro* models, it will be hard to justify human trials with combinations until a single trophic factor is successful.

Some of the issues of bioavailability may be overcome by development of small non-peptide agents which affect the release or activation of growth factors (e.g. xaliproden, above) or by the designer molecule approach, in which short amino acid sequences that bind to trophic factor receptor active sites are used to increase bioavailability or mitigate antibody production (e.g. PEDF, above). Still more futuristic aspects of the pharmacotherapy of the motor neuron disorders are explored in detail in Chapter 9.

References

ALS CNTF Treatment Study Group (1996) A double-blind placebo-controlled clinical trial of subcutaneous recombinant human ciliary neurotrophic factor (rHCNTF) in amyotrophic lateral sclerosis. Neurology 46: 1244–1249.

Altar CA, Cai N, Bliven T et al. (1997) Anterograde transport of brain-derived neurotrophic factor and its role in the brain. Nature 389: 856–860.

Appel SH, Smith RG, Alexianu MF, Engelhardt JI, Stefani E (1995) Autoimmunity as an etiological factor in sporadic amyotrophic lateral sclerosis. Adv Neurol. 68: 47–57.

Askmark H, Aquilonius SM, Gillberg PG, Liedhom LJ, Stalberg E, Wuopio R (1993) A pilot trial of dextromethorphan in amyotrophic lateral sclerosis. J Neurol Neurosurg Psych 56: 197–200.

Bensimon G, Lacomblez L, Meininger V, The ALS/Riluzole Study Group (1994) A controlled trial of riluzole in amyotrophic lateral sclerosis. N Engl J Med 330: 585–591.

Bernstein K (1997) BioCentury 5, A1–A2.

Bilak MM, Corse AM, Bilak SR, Lehar M, Tombran-Tink J, Kuncl RW (1999a) Pigment epithelium-derived factor (PEDF) protects motor neurons from chronic glutamate-mediated neurodegeneration. J Neuropath Exp Neurol 58: 719–728.

Bilak MM, Shifrin DA, Corse AM, Bilak SR, Kuncl RW (1999b) Neuroprotective utility and neurotrophic action of neurturin in postnatal motor neurons: comparison with GDNF and persephin. Mol Cell Neurosci 13: 326–336.

Bilak MM, Corse AM, Becerra P, Kuncl RW (1999c) A small peptide from human pigment epithelium-derived factor protects motor neurons from chronic glutamate-mediated degeneration. Soc Neurosci Abst 25: 1108.

Bilak MM, Corse AM, Kuncl RW (2001a) Additivity and potentiation of IGF-1 and GDNF in the complete rescue of postnatal motor neurons. ALS Other Motor Neuron Dis 2: 83–91.

Bilak MM, Becerra SP, Moss BH et al. (2001b) Mechanisms for motor neuron protection by pigment epithelium-derived factor: evidence for the presence of PEDF receptors on motor neurons. Soc Neurosci Abst 27: Program No. 97.16.

Bilak MM, Kuncl RW (2001) Delayed application of IGF-1 and GDNF can rescue already injured postnatal motor neurons. Neuroreport 12: 2531–2535.

Blin O, Pouget J, Aubrespy G, Guelton C, Crevat A, Serratrice G (1992) A double-blind placebo-controlled trial of L-threonine in amyotrophic lateral sclerosis. J Neurol 239: 79–81.

Blin O, Azulay JP, Desnuelle C et al. (1996) A controlled one-year trial of dextromethorphan in amyotrophic lateral sclerosis. Clin Neuropharmacol 19(2): 189–192.

Borasio GD, Robberecht W, Leigh PN et al. (1998) A placebo-controlled trial of insulin-like growth factor-I in amyotrophic lateral scterosis. Neurology 51: 583–586.

Brodie MJ (1992) Drug profiles: lamotrigine. Lancet 339: 397–1400.

Cedarbaum JM, Stambler N, Brooks BR, Bradley W (1998) Brain-derived neurotrophic factor in amyotrophic lateral sclerosis: a failed drug or a failed trial. Ann Neurol 44: 506–507.

Chan JM, Stampfer MJ, Giovannucci E et al. (1998) Plasma insulin-like growth factor-I and prostate cancer risk: a prospective study. Science 279: 563–566.

Choi DW (1988) Glutamate neurotoxicity and diseases of the nervous system. Neuron 1: 623–634.

Chou SM, Harman HA (1964) Axonal lesions and waltzing syndrome after IDPN administration in rats. Acta Neuropathol (Berl) 4: 428–450.

Conover JC, Erickson JT, Katz DM et al. (1995) Neuronal deficits, not involving motor neurons, in mice lacking BDNF and/or NT4. Nature 375: 235–238.

Cork LC, Griffin JW, Munnell JF et al. (1979) Hereditary canine spinal muscular atrophy. J Neuropathol Exp Neurol 38: 209–221.

Corse AM, Bilak MM, Bilak SR, Lehar M, Rothstein JD, Kuncl RW (1999) Preclinical testing of neuroprotective neurotrophic factors in a model of chronic motor neuron degeneration. Neurobiol Dis 6: 335–346.

Côte F, Collard J-F, Julien J-P (1993) Progressive neuronopathy in transgenic mice expressing the human neurofilament heavy gene: a mouse model of amyotrophic lateral sclerosis. Cell 73: 35–46.

Couratier P, Hugon J, Sindou P, Vallat JM, Dumas M (1993) Cell culture evidence for neuronal degeneration in amyotrophic lateral sclerosis being linked to glutamate AMPA/Kainate receptors. Lancet 341: 265–268.

Couratier P, Sindou P, Esclaire F, Louvel E, Hugon J (1994) Neuroprotective effects of riluzole in ALS CSF toxicity. Neuroreport 5: 1012–1014.

Curtis R, Adryan KM, Zhu Y et al. (1993) Retrograde axonal transport of ciliary neurotrophic factor is increased by peripheral nerve injury. Nature 365: 253–255.

Dittrich F, Thoenen H, Sendtner M (1994) Ciliary neurotrophic factor: Pharmacokinetics and acute phase response in rat. Ann Neurol 35: 151–163.

Dittrich F, Ochs G, Grosse-Wilde A et al. (1996) Pharmacokinetics of intrathecally applied BDNF and effects on spinal motoneurons. Exp Neurol 141: 225–239.

Doble A (1996) The pharmacology and mechanism of action of riluzole. Neurology 47 (suppl 4): S233–S241.

Duong F, Fournier J, Keane PE et al. (1998) The effect of the nonpeptide neurotrophic compound SR 57746A on the progression of the disease state of the pmn mouse. Br J Pharmacol 124: 811–817.

Eisen A, Stewart H, Schulzer M, Cameron D (1993) Anti-glutamate therapy in amyotrophic lateral sclerosis: a trial using lamotrigine. Can J Neurol Sci 20(4): 297–301.

Fournier J, Steinberg R, Gauthier T et al. (1993) Protective effects of SR57746A in central and peripheral models of neurodegenerative disorders in rodents and primates. Neuroscience 55: 629–641.

Fournier J, Boutot G, Keane PE, Maffrand JP, Le Fur G, Soubrie P (1998) The non-peptide neuroprotective agent SR 57746A interacts with neurotrophin 3 to induce differentiation in the PC12 cell-line. J Pharm Pharmacol 50: 323–327.

Gravel C, Gütz R, Lorrain A, Sendtner M (1997) Adenoviral gene transfer of ciliary neurotrophic factor and brain-derived neurotrophic factor leads to long-term survival of axotomized motor neurons. Nature Med 3: 765–770.

Gredal O, Werdelin L, Bak S et al. (1997) A clinical trial of dextromethorphan in amyotrophic lateral sclerosis. Acta Neurol Scand 96(1): 8–13.

Gurney ME, Pu H, Chiu AY et al. (1994) Motor neuron degeneration in mice that express a human Cu,Zn superoxide dismutase mutation. Science 264: 1772–1775.

Gurney ME, Cutting FB, Zhai P et al. (1996) Benefit of vitamin E, riluzole, and gabapentin in a transgenic model of familial amyotrophic lateral sclerosis. Ann Neurol 39(2): 147–157.

Haase G, Kennel P, Pettmann B et al. (1997) Gene therapy of murine motor neuron disease using adenoviral vectors for neurotrophic factors. Nature Med 3: 429–436.

Hefti F (1997) Pharmacology of neurotrophic factors. Annu Rev Pharmacol Toxicol 37: 239–267.

Hugon J, Tabaraud F, Rigaud M, Vallat JM, Dumas M (1989) Glutamate dehydrogenase (GDH) and asparatate aminotransferase (AAT) in leucocytes of patients with motoneuron disease. Neurology 39: 956–958.

Hugon J, Ludolph A, Roy DN, Schaumburg HH, Spencer PS (1988) Studies on the etiology and pathogenesis of motor neuron diseases. II. Clinical and electrophysiologic features of pyramidal dysfunction in macaques fed lathyrus sativus and IDPN. Neurology 38: 435–442.

Hugon J, Vallat J-M, Spencer PS, Leboutet M-J, Barthe D (1989) Kainic acid induces acute and delayed neuronal damages in rat spinal cord. Neurosci Lett 104: 758–763.

Hugon J, Preux PM, Gremy C et al. (1992) Glycine and L-threonine therapeutic trials in amyotrophic lateral sclerosis (ALS). Neurology 42: 454.

Ikeda K, Klinkosz B, Greene T et al. (1995) Effects of brain-derived neurotrophic factor on motor dysfunction in wobbler mouse motor neuron disease. Ann Neurol 37: 505–511.

Jossan SS, Ekblom J, Gudjonsson O, Hagbarth KE, Aquilonius SM (1994) Double blind cross over trial with deprenyl in amyotrophic lateral sclerosis. J Neural Transm Suppl 41: 237–241.

Klivenyi P, Ferrante RJ, Matthews RT et al. (1999) Neuroprotective effects of creatine in a transgenic animal model of amyotrophic lateral sclerosis. Nature Med 5: 347–350.

Koh IY, Gwag BJ, Lobner D, Choi DW (1995) Potentiated necrosis of cultured cortical neurons by neurotrophins. Science 268: 573–575.

Kostic V, Jackson-Lewis V, de Bilbao F, Dubois-Dauphin M, Przedborski S (1997) Bcl-2: Prolonging life in a transgenic mouse model of familial amyotrophic lateral sclerosis. Science 277: 559–562.

Lacomblez L, Bensimon G, Leigh PN, Guillet P, Meininger V, for the amyotrophic lateral sclerosis/riluzole study group II. (1996) Dose-ranging study of riluzole in amyotrophic lateral sclerosis. Lancet 347: 1425–1431.

Lai EC, Felice KJ, Festoff BW et al. and the North America ALS/IGF-1 Study Group (1997) Effect of recombinant human insulin-like growth factor-I on progression of ALS. Neurology 49: 1621–1630.

Lange DJ (1996) Recombinant human IGF-1 in ALS: description of a double blind-placebo controlled study. North American ALS/IGF-1 study group. Neurology 47 (Suppl. 2): S93–S95.

Lange DJ, Murphy PL, Diamond B, Appel V, Lai EC, Younger DS, Appel SH (1998) Selegiline is ineffective in a collaborative double-blind, placebo-controlled trial for treatment of amyotrophic lateral sclerosis. Arch Neurol 55(1): 93–96.

Langston JW (1990) Selegiline as neuroprotective therapy in Parkinson's disease: concepts and controversies. Neurology 40(10 suppl 3): 61–66.

Le Roith D (1997) Insulin-like growth factors. N Engl J Med 336: 633–640.

Leigh PN, The North American and European ALS/IGF-1 Study Groups (1997) The treatment of ALS with recombinant human insulin-like growth factor I (rhIGF-1): Pooled analysis of two clinical trials. Neurology 48(suppl 3): A217–A218.

Leist M, Nicotera P (1998) Apoptosis, excitotoxicity, and neuropathology. Exp Cell Res 239(2): 183–201.

Li M, Ona VO, Guégan C et al. (2000) Functional role of caspase-1 and caspase-3 in an ALS transgenic mouse model. Science 288: 283–284.

Lin LF, Doherty DH, Lile JD, Bektesh S, Collins F (1993) GDNF: a glial cell line-derived neurotropic factor for midbrain dopaminergic neurons. Science 260: 1130–1132.

Louvel E, Hugon J, Doble A (1997) Therapeutic advances in amyotrophic lateral sclerosis. Trends Pharmacol Sci 18: 196–203.

Louwerse ES, Weverling GJ, Bossuyt PMM, Meyjes FEP, de Jong JMBV (1995) Randomized, double-blind, controlled trial of acetylcysteine in amyotrophic lateral sclerosis. Arch Neurol 52: 559–564.

Ludolph A, Hugon J, Dwivedi MP, Schaumburg HH, Spencer PS (1987) Studies on the etiology and pathogenesis of motor neuron diseases. Lathyrism: clinical findings in established cases. Brain 110: 149–165.

Ludolph AC (1996) Animal models for motor neuron diseases: Research directions. Neurology 47(4): S228–S232.

Maher T, Wurtman RJ (1980) L-threonine administration increases glycine concentration in the rat central nervous system. Life Sci 26: 1283–1286.

Martin LJ (1999) Neuronal death in amyotrophic lateral sclerosis is apoptosis: possible contribution of a programmed cell death mechanism. J Neuropathol Exp Neurol 58: 459–471.

Martin LJ (2000) p53 is abnormally elevated and active in the CNS of patients with amyotrophic lateral sclerosis. Neurobiol Dis 7: 613–622.

Matthews RT, Yang L, Browne S, Baik M, Beal MF (1998) Coenzyme Q10 administration increases brain mitochondrial concentrations and exerts neuroprotective effects. Proc Natl Acad Sci USA 95: 8892–8897.

Mazzini L, Testa D, Balzarini C, Mora G (1994) An open-randomized clinical trial of selegiline in amyotrophic lateral sclerosis. J Neurol 241(4): 223–227.

Messer A, Flaherty L (1986) Autosomal dominance in a late onset motor neuron disease in the mouse. J Neurogenet 3: 345–355.

Milbrandt J, Sauvage FJ, Fahrner TJ, et al. (1998) Persephin, a novel neurotrophic factor related to GDNF and neurturin. Neuron 20: 245–253.

Miller RG, Bryan WW, Dietz MA et al. (1996a) Toxicity and tolerability of recombinant human ciliary neurotrophic factor in patients with amyotrophic lateral sclerosis. Neurology 47: 1329–1331.

Miller RG, Moore D, Young LA et al. (1996b) Placebo-controlled trial of gabapentin in patients with amyotrophic lateral sclerosis. Neurology, 47: 1383–1388.

Miller RG, Petajan JH, Bryan WW et al. and the rhCNTF ALS Study Group (1996c) A placebo-controlled trial of recombinant human ciliary neurotrophic (rhCNTF) factor in amyotrophic lateral sclerosis. Ann Neurol 39: 256–260.

Miller RG, Shepherd R, Dao H et al. (1996d) Controlled trial of nimodipine in amyotrophic lateral sclerosis. Neuromusc Disord 6(2): 101–104.

Miller RG, Smith SA, Murphy JR et al. (1996e) A clinical trial of verapamil in amyotrophic lateral sclerosis. Muscle Nerve 19(4): 511–515.

Miller RG, Moore DH, Gelinas DF, Dronsky V, Mendoza M et al. (2001) Phase III randomized trial of gabapentin in patients with amyotrophic lateral sclerosis. Neurology 56: 843–848.

Mitsumoto H, Pioro EP (1995) Animal models of amyotrophic lateral sclerosis. Adv Neurol 68: 73–87.

Mitsumoto H, Ikeda K, Klinkosz B, Cedarbaum JM, Wong V, Lindsay RM (1994) Arrest of motor neuron disease in wobbler mice cotreated with CNTF and BDNF. Science 265: 1107–1110.

Mitsumoto H, Tsuzaka K (1999a) Neurotrophic factors and neuromuscular disease: I. General comments, the neurotrophin family, and neuropoietic cytokines. Muscle Nerve 22: 983–999.

Mitsumoto H, Tsuzaka K (1999b) Neurotrophic factors and neuromuscular disease: II. GDNF, other neurotrophic factors, and future directions. Muscle Nerve 22: 1000–1021.

Nader R, Growdon JH, Mahre TJ, Wurtman RJ (1987) L-threonine administration increases CSF glycine levels and suppresses spasticity. Neurology 37: 125.

Neff NT, Prevette D, Houenou LJ, et al. (1993) Insulin-like growth factors: putative muscle-derived trophic agents that promote motoneuron survival. J Neurobiol 24(12): 1578–1588.

Ochs G, Penn RD, Beck M et al. (1998) Intrathecal infusion of recombinant met-human-brain-derived neurotrophic factor (rhBDNF) is well tolerated in patients with ALS. Abstract, 9th International symposium on ALS/MND.

Oppenheim RW, Houenou LJ, Johnson JE, et al. (1995) Developing motor neurons rescued from programmed and axotomy-induced cell death by GDNF. Nature 373: 344–346.

Patten BM, Houston TX, Lynn MK (1988) L-threonine and the modification of ALS. Neurology 38: 354–355.

Penn RD, Kroin JS, York MM, Cedarbaum JM (1997) Intrathecal ciliary neurotrophic factor delivery for treatment of amyotrophic lateral sclerosis (phase I trial). Neurosurgery 40: 94–99.

Plaitakis A, Caroscio JT (1987) Abnormal glutamate metabolism in amyotrophic lateral sclerosis. Ann Neurol 22: 575–579.

Plaitakis A, Smith J, Mandell J, Yahr MD (1988) Pilot trial of branched-chain aminoacids in amyotrophic lateral sclerosis. Lancet 1(8593): 1015–1018.

Poduslo JF, Curran GL (1996) Permeability at the blood–brain and blood–nerve barriers of the neurotrophic factors NGF, CNTF, NT-3, BDNF. Brain Res Mol Brain Res 36: 280–286.

Rothstein JD, Kuncl RW (1995) Neuroprotective strategies in a model of chronic glutamate-mediated motor neuron toxicity. J Neurochem 65: 643–651.

Rothstein JD, Tsai, Kuncl RW (1990) Abnormal excitatory aminoacid metabolism in amyotrophic lateral sclerosis. Ann Neurol 28: 18–25.

Rothstein JD, Martin LJ, Kuncl RW (1992) Decreased glutamate transport by the brain and spinal cord in amyotrophic lateral sclerosis. N Engl J Med 326: 1464–1468.

Rothstein JD, Jin L, Dykes-Hoberg M, Kuncl RW (1993) Chronic inhibition of glutamate uptake produces a model of slow neurotoxicity. Proc Natl Acad Sci USA 90: 6591–6595.

Rothstein JD, Van Kammen M, Levey AI, Martin L, Kuncl RW (1995) Selective loss of glial glutamate transporter GLT-1 in amyotrophic lateral sclerosis. Ann Neurol 38: 73–84.

Sagot Y, Tan SA, Baetge E et al. (1995) Polymer encapsulated cell lines genetically engineered to release recombinant ciliary neurotrophic factor can slow down progressive motor neuropathy in the mouse. Eur J Neurosci 7: 1313–1322.

Schmalbruch H, Jensen H-JS, Bjaerg M et al (1991) A new mouse mutant with progressive motor neuronopathy. J Neuropathol Exp Neurol 50: 192–204.

Sendtner M (1997) Gene therapy for motor neuron disease. Nature Med 3: 380–381.

Sendtner M, Kreutzberg GW, Thoenen H (1990) Ciliary neurotrophic factor prevents the degeneration of motor neurons after axotomy. Nature 345: 440–441.

Sendtner M, Schmalbruch H, Stockli KA et al. (1992) Ciliary neurotrophic factor prevents degeneration of motor neurons in mouse mutant progressive motor neuronopathy. Nature 358: 502–504.

Smith RA, Melmed S, Sherman B, Frane J, Munsat TL, Festoff BW (1993) Recombinant growth factor treatment of amyotrophic lateral sclerosis. Muscle Nerve 16: 624–633.

Spencer PS, Roy DN, Ludolph AC, Hugon J, Dwivedi MP, Schaumburg HH (1986) Lathyrism: evidence for role of the neuroexcitatory amino acid BOAA. Lancet 2(8515): 1066–1067.

Spencer PS, Nunn PB, Hugon J et al. (1987) Guam amyotrophic lateral sclerosis-parkinsonism-dementia linked to a plant excitant neurotoxin. Science, 237: 517–522.

Steinberg GK (1991) Effects of dextromethorphan on regional cerebral blood flow in focal cerebral ischemia. J Cereb Blood Flow Metab 11: 803–809.

Tarnopolsky MA, Beal MF (2001) Potential for creatine and other therapies targeting cellular energy dysfunction in neurological disorders. Ann Neurol 49: 561–574.

Testa D, Caraceni T, FeToni V (1989) Branched-chain amino acids in the treatment of amyotrophic lateral sclerosis. J Neurol 236: 445–447.

Vaught JL, Contreras PC, Glicksman MA, Neff NT (1996) Potential utility of rhIGF-1 in neuromuscular and/or degenerative disease. In: Growth Factors as Drugs for Neurological and Sensory Disorders (Ciba Foundation Symposium 196). Wiley; Chichester, pp. 18–38.

Walter MC, Lochmuller H, Reilich P, (2000) Creatine monohydrate in muscular dystrophies: A double-blind, placebo-controlled clinical study. Neurology 54: 1848–1850.

Wong B, Coulter D, Choi D, Priner D (1987) Dextrorphan and dextromethorphan, common antitussives, are antiepileptic and antagonize NMDA in brain slices. Soc Neurosci Abstr 13: 1560.

Wong PC, Pardo CA, Borchelt DR et al. (1995) An adverse property of a familial ALS-linked SOD1 mutation causes motor neuron disease characterized by vacuolar degeneration of mitochondria. Neuron 14: 1105–1116.

Yan Q, Matheson C, Lopez OT (1995) In vivo neurotrophic effects of GDNF on neonatal and adult facial motor neurons. Nature 373: 341–344.

Zorumski CF, Olney JW (1993) Excitotoxic neuronal damage and neuropsychiatric disorders. Pharmacol Ther 59(2): 145–162.

Zurn AD, Baetge EE, Hammang JP, Tan SA, Aebischer P (1994) Glial cell line-derived neurotrophic factor, a new neurotrophic factor for motoneurons. NeuroReport 6: 113–118.

CHAPTER 7

Multidisciplinary approach to management and support of patients

Judith Richman and Patricia Casey

The multidisciplinary team approach to the management and support of patients with amyotrophic lateral sclerosis (ALS) makes use of several branches of knowledge developed to care for these complex patients. In the United States, the multidisciplinary team approach was first formalized after World War II in VA hospitals and private state rehabilitation facilities. The many needs of patients who had suffered cataclysmic war injuries, both physical and psychological, had to be addressed. Tuberculosis sanatoriums had long appreciated the roles of the developing medical specialties in promoting healing and independence in patients with long-term conditions. The multidisciplinary team has been successfully used in rehabilitation, psychiatric, and children's hospitals as well as in the management of acute poliomyelitis. ALS, however, is a chronic condition usually contracted by persons who have 'never been sick before' and who will usually have no need for inpatient hospitalizations, except for the acute care of pulmonary infections or gastrostomy placement.

Current healthcare systems throughout the world demand less expensive, short-term, outpatient care with as few physician and medical specialty visits as possible. Yet patients with ALS are some of the neediest patients seen in practice. Even though most ALS teams consist of professionals who are not employed full-time to care solely for ALS patients, they should be knowledgeable and committed to this patient population to guarantee quality care and continuity of treatment. Patients desire access to the most up-to-date treatment. The physician needs a shared team approach to care for patients, even in these cost-cutting health management times.

More and more, the idea of employing a multidisciplinary approach is well accepted, but the interpretation and use of this approach varies among individual healthcare professionals and settings. Within a large university ALS specialty clinic, the multidisciplinary approach is generally recognized as the best means to support this patient population. Here there is the recognition that giving the diagnosis of ALS does not mean 'go home and get your affairs in order; you have a couple of years to live'. Rather, referrals are made to those who recognize that patients with ALS are treatable and the team has the resources to help. Alternatively, physicians who do not have access to a support team must be knowledgeable about ALS and what other disciplines can offer their patients.

Since ALS is a devastating disease for which there is no known cure, one may ask why the team approach is so important. Patients and their families need to draw upon every available resource to help them live with this disease and bring quality to their lives. The multidisciplinary team is this resource.

The 'basic team' may employ as many as eight disciplines, including neurologist, nurse specialist, occupational therapist (OT), social worker, physical therapist (PT), pulmonologist, speech pathologist, and nutritionist. The patient and primary caregiver are also considered integral members of the team. In this chapter, we concentrate on the medical professional team. Having these disciplines involved in the care of the patient on site is ideal, but in some settings this may be infeasible or financially impractical. Patients need to be comfortable, not only with their physician, but also with the others involved in their care. Many patients state that it is too overwhelming to be seen by numerous people and do not want to feel as if they are being treated on an 'assembly line'. Our goal is to avoid this, and so we create a 'primary team' which includes the neurologist, nurse, OT and social worker. The physician and nurse draw upon their expertise to direct the rest of the team.

The team has a responsibility to provide patients and their caregivers with as much information as possible to help them cope with this disease. It is our philosophy not to dwell on the fact that a cure does not exist at this time. Instead, we focus on what we, as healthcare professionals, can do to help our patients. It is our responsibility as specialists to address our patients' need for knowledge and understanding of the disease, to manage their symptoms, to provide appropriate therapies, to address issues regarding breathing, diet, nutrition, communication, swallowing, and above all to manage the psychosocial problems.

This chapter will review and summarize the roles of each member of the multidisciplinary team. We will examine how we support our patients and manage symptomatic care when there is 'nothing to do'. In reality, there is plenty to do.

Physician's role

The physician and nurse direct the team. They must be well versed in all areas of patient care and should work in conjunction to provide the best overall care. As the patient's condition changes, they should determine when to introduce other team members or make referrals to disciplines outside the team. However, there is one responsibility that falls solely on the physician's shoulders: giving the diagnosis.

Confirming the diagnosis of ALS is never easy. The diagnosis should not be given quickly, whether a patient is being seen for an initial evaluation or second opinion. Therefore, the physician should explain that a complete battery of tests and procedures will be performed in order to rule out any other condition that may mimic ALS. It is preferable to complete the testing in a timely manner, then meet a second time with patient, family and significant others to discuss the results and diagnosis. The ideal time frame for this process should be within one month of the initial visit. Due to the devastating nature of this discussion, it is best to conduct this meeting in an unhurried manner without any interruptions. It is the physician's responsibility to explain the disease process, prognosis, and treatment options in language patients can understand and in a compassionate yet authoritative manner. The physician must be able to provide information regarding current research, available clinical trials and, above all, convey the idea that there is hope throughout the course of the disease process. While providers cannot cure ALS, we can offer and provide treatment to help ease the burden, both for the patient and the caregivers. Above all, they must understand that they are not alone in struggling with the day-to-day frustrations and burdens of living with ALS.

Once the diagnosis has been given, it is advisable to see the patient on a regular basis. Depending on the patient's condition, these follow-up visits should be every 2–3 months in order to assess ongoing physical and psychosocial needs. As the disease progresses, the physician must be able to judge when it is best to discuss the problems of swallowing, breathing, and end-of-life issues. Although no one wants to confront their own mortality, it is necessary to bring these issues to light so that the patient's family never needs to say, 'why didn't you tell us this?' Discussions regarding feeding tubes, ventilatory assistance and hospice must be open and honest; however, the physician must be sensitive to how much information the patient and caregivers are able to absorb at each visit. Patients and their caregivers will hear only what they want to hear at their own pace. Therefore, most discussions will need to be reinforced on a periodic basis.

Symptom management is an ongoing process. Although medications are available and readily prescribed for any number of symptoms (see Table 7.1), physicians must also be attuned to utilizing other disciplines and other means in management. Now the team approach comes into play, with one of the key players being the ALS nurse specialist.

Table 7.1 Symptom management approaches

Overall disease	ALS team expertise, Riluzole
Muscle weakness/fatigue	OT, PT, speech pathologist, Pyridostigmine bromide
Spasticity	Baclofen, tizanidine HCl, clonazepam
Muscle cramps	Quinine sulfate, diazepam, gabapentin, magnesium oxide
Sialorrhea	Amitriptyline, diphenhydramine HCl, scopalamine patch, glycopyrrolate, propantheline bromide, SSKI, suction machine
Phlegm	Fluid intake, guaifenesin, papase
Sleep disturbance	Amitriptyline, zolpidem tartrate, diphenhydramine HCl, clonazepam, positioning
Dyspnea	Relaxation/breathing exercises, low-flow oxygen, pulmonary consult, BiPap, nebulizer, morphine/Roxanol
Pain/discomfort	Relafen, ibuprofen, positioning, cushions, exercise
Constipation	Fluid intake, increased fiber, exercise program, stool softeners, laxatives such as Senokot, enemas if needed
Emotional lability	Amitriptyline
Depression	Sertraline HCl, venlafaxine HCl, paroxetine, amitriptyline, counseling
Nutrition/weight loss	Vitamins E and C, nutritional supplements, nutritional consult, feeding tubes
End-of-life issues	Advanced directive, ventilation with tracheostomy, oxygen, hospice, home care, nursing care facility

Nurse's role

If you were to ask ALS nurses what they do, in all likelihood the response would be, 'just about everything'. In most specialty clinic settings, nurses play a pivotal role. They are part of the 'team within a team' and in most instances are the primary contact for patients and carers.

The ALS nurse usually is the one who oversees the day-to-day management and care issues that arise. It is preferable to have a nurse with a background in neurology, and ideally one who specializes in motor neuron disease/ALS. Neurology patients have special needs, and the nurse must be able to incorporate knowledge of the pathophysiology of ALS with basic nursing skills in order to meet those needs. The nurse must also be able to incorporate chronic care and rehabilitation skills. He or she should also know about and be able to implement services that other disciplines can provide for this patient population. In many instances, the role of the ALS nurse takes on some of the aspects of the OT, PT, nutritionist, pulmonologist, speech therapist and social worker.

Depending on how each clinic or practice operates, the nurse is often the first person a patient and family has contact with, either by phone or in person. From that time on, a unique relationship usually develops among the patient, family members, and nurse. In most instances, these patients have never been sick and have no idea what is in store. Once again, it must be conveyed to patients and their families that they are not alone to fend for themselves in coping with this devastating disease. From the time of the initial visit, the nurse should be available to patients and family members for clarification of information, answers and guidance. Since every day can present a new problem, much of the help our patients need is managed through phone calls.

One of the nurse's most important functions is performing a needs assessment with each patient contact. Questions regarding eating, dressing, bathing, toileting, sleeping, social activities, work, family situation, emotional health, support systems, and medications are reviewed. Once the physician and nurse discuss this information, a plan of care is formulated and implemented. As the disease progresses and the patients' needs change, the care plan must be constantly updated based upon the ongoing assessments by the physician and the nurse. It is the nurse's role to introduce the services of other disciplines when appropriate.

Patient teaching has always been a key nursing function. From the time the diagnosis of ALS is even mentioned, patients, family members and friends start to gather pertinent information about the disease. Patients usually fall into three categories: active, passive, or benign neglect. Those who actively seek information obtain all the brochures available, purchase the ALS Association (ALSA) manuals, surf the Internet, etc., even before a final diagnosis is given. They devour any and all information that is available on ALS. Those who passively obtain information assimilate bits and pieces given to them from others, usually well-meaning friends. They will eventually accept and order ALS pamphlets, but they are not in a hurry to obtain the information. Then there are those in the benign neglect category. These patients rely solely on the healthcare team for information. This group wants to know only what they need to know at the present.

As mentioned earlier, one of the physician's responsibilities is to discuss the disease process, treatment options and prognosis. But early on, patients are in a state of disbelief over the diagnosis of ALS. They not only do not hear everything discussed but cannot absorb much of the information given to them. People learn in different stages, making ongoing patient education one of the most important roles for the ALS nurse. We find it beneficial to reinforce to the patient and family members that we do not expect them to understand, nor should they try to, everything about ALS all at once. We encourage them to call us in order to clarify *any* information they receive, whether the source is the office visit, books, newspapers, magazine articles, or *especially* the Internet.

Depending on the level of care needed, the physician and nurse can provide answers and help. However, they must recognize when the type of care required is beyond their areas of expertise and referrals should be made to other team members.

Finally, one of the most important nursing functions is to act as a patient advocate. Depending on a country's healthcare system, the extent of this function varies. In the United States, insurance companies and managed care organizations often dictate whether adaptive equipment, physical therapy, home care, specialty referrals, tests and procedures, or hospice are warranted. Often those making the decision have no knowledge of ALS. Therefore, nurses must combine the role of educator and patient advocate by writing letters of medical necessity.

Indeed, the role of ALS nurses is diverse. They formulate and implement a plan of care, educate patients and caregivers as well as the general public, direct patient care and, above all, provide emotional support.

Occupational therapist's role

The occupational therapist (OT) promotes independence in activities of daily living (ADL). These include self-care and work activities. Because ALS is a progressive disease, selection of assistive devices and alternate methods of performing ADL is a continuous process. The patient's perspective counts most. Intervention is determined according to those symptoms which are the patient's priorities. Assessment of the primary caregiver's strengths and abilities are given equal consideration when recommendations are made. The therapist evaluates what importance each activity holds, the patient's physical ability and willingness to change, and what burden is placed on the caregiver. Good suggestions may be of little help if the patient is not concerned about performing a certain activity independently. On the other hand, a caregiver may be unwilling or physically unable to help the patient. The family may not be able to purchase the expensive equipment that would allow independence. The OT helps prescribe appropriate assistive equipment with consideration of the patient's idea of independence. A more difficult task is helping patients consider alternatives without discouraging or unnecessarily depressing them in case a regimen of therapy does not work. A practical rule is that no one changes their way of doing things unless it becomes absolutely necessary. This varies from person to person; the same good idea does not work for everyone who has a similar problem. Conversely, a patient's need to deny the progression of symptoms because 'I'm not that bad yet' must also be considered. Recommendations must be individualized and a course of treatment initiated according to each person's need to remain independent.

The patient's and caregiver's abilities can be assessed in two settings, the clinic and home. The patient can answer questions regarding dressing, toileting, grooming, hygiene and bathing skills in the clinic and can demonstrate how some of these activities are performed. However, important considerations for assistive equipment, wheelchairs and energy-saving techniques that may help both patient and caregiver may be underassessed if questions about placement of furniture, layout of home and garage, (especially bathrooms, stairways, and exits) are not asked. Home visits are needed to determine where obstacles impede safe ambulation or wheelchair use. Typical obstacles include depth of carpeting and padding, thresholds, throw rugs, width of doorways and hallways, radius needed for corner turns, configuration of bathroom layout, presence of bathtub/shower stall with or without glass sliding doors, stairway placement with/without rails, entrances/exits, porches, decks, garages and driveways. Even the arrangement of bedroom furniture and the spouses' preferred side of the bed are sometimes difficult mobility issues.

Recommendations for various assistive devices depend on areas of weakness and are summarized in Table 7.2–7.5.

Social worker's role

At some point in the course of the disease process, all of our patients and families have emotional and psychosocial needs to be addressed. Patients and families experience changes in their roles, responsibilities and relationships as the disease progresses. A social worker not only helps provide the emotional support and counseling but also manages access to valuable community resources.

The social worker should meet with the patient and significant others at either the initial or second clinic visit. However, the degree and timing of intervention varies according to the family's 'comfort zone' in talking openly to a stranger. Every person will react to the diagnosis of ALS differently. Some of the basic behaviors patients exhibit are anger, denial, depression, dependency struggle, and despair. Family members may become angry or disappointed, especially in the case of newly (re)married couples. Healthcare professionals must assess patients' previous coping mechanisms in order to help them manage the road ahead. We collect as much background information as possible, such as identification of the primary caregiver, types of support systems in place, previous response to illness, employment/financial status, insurance coverage, family dynamics, and religious beliefs. The social worker

Table 7.2 Assistive devices for upper extremity weakness

Eating	Foam tubing to build up eating utensils or heavy-duty plastic dinnerware Elastic utensil holder Large-handled plastic lightweight mug Plateguard or rimmed plate Rocker knife Jar openers with leverage handle Extra-long reusable plastic straws Wheelchair beverage holder Nonskid mat (Dycem) Mobile arm supports with table mount clamps, T-bar and supinator attachments Adjustable-height overbed table on gliders/wheels with tilt top
Personal hygiene/grooming	Foam tubing for razor handle, toothbrush, nail file Floss holders Electric toothbrush with rotary brush Large-handled comb Hairbrush with velcro strap Large-handled nailclippers Nail brush/clippers on suction cups Hand-held shower hose Push-button soap dispenser for shampoo, soap, cream rinse, lotion (suction device for shower/bathtub wall) Toilet paper tongs to use with paper or baby wipes Faucet levers instead of knobs
Dressing	Large-handled button hooks Zipper pulls (paper clips or fish line loops may do) Velcro clothing closures Pullover shirts and pants with knit, polyester or nylon content Pull-on pants with elastic waistbands Suspenders Long-handled shoehorn Reachers with trigger or quad lever
Recreation/Leisure	Key holder Self-opening scissors Book holder, overbed tilt-top table, lap table with pillow positioner Doorknob adaptors Touch switch for lamps Extension knob for light switches Knob turner
Communication	Speaker phone with speed dial Portable headphone Triangular or foam tubing on pencil Hand clip for phone TTD (Telecommunications Device for the Deaf) for phone (relays phone messages through the operator)
Positioning	Elastic wrist supports for wear during the day Plastic lightweight hand/wrist positional splints to wear at night or during the day to reduce or prevent wrist and finger contracture (instruct patient to wear only one splint at a time to allow use of other hand) Index finger spiral splint

makes appropriate recommendations as the needs of the patient and caregiver change.

A patient usually turns to family members and friends for support, but they may not always be up to the task. Some patients, usually men, while maintaining their position as head of the household, try to protect family members by claiming

Table 7.3 Assistive devices and durable medical equipment for lower extremity weakness

Ankle/foot weakness	
	Straight cane with large rubber tip
	Two canes or forearm crutches for weak or spastic gait
	Plastic ankle-foot orthoses for foot drop with articulating ankles if stairclimbing necessary at home or work (5–10° plantar flexion for weak knee extension)
Hip weakness	
	Gait belt
	Transfer board (some have rolling seat disk for easy bed/car transfer)
	Rolling walker with hand brakes and seat
	Seat lift recliner chair
	Fully electric hospital bed which rises from the floor and assists the person to a standing position
	Raised toilet seat with attached side rails
	Tub rail or grab bars in tub/shower area
	Barstool in shower area
	Padded bathtub bench or seat, with a back and adjustable-height legs
	Rolling commode/shower chairs with removable or drop-arm feature and secure wheel brakes
	Hydraulic patient lifts with heavy duty separating slings (extra length for head and neck support)
	Wheelchairs: manual for transportation; power for independent mobility
	Stairlifts for two-story or bi- and tri-level homes
	Porch lifts or ramps
	Vans with wheelchair lift

Table 7.4 Assistive devices and durable medical equipment for trunk/neck weakness

High back support on armchairs, bath chairs, wheelchairs
Head and neck supports (cervical pillows, foam cervical collars or wire orthoses – whatever is most comfortable)
Headrest supports attached to wheelchair or shower chair
Head straps attached to high back recliner or wheelchair headrest attachment
Tilt-in-space seating feature on wheelchair frame
Trunk positioning aids (contoured wheelchair seating, foam supports to position the arms while sitting, body pillows for positioning while sleeping

Table 7.5 Assistive devices and durable medical equipment for speech/swallowing weakness

Mouth hygiene aids (lemon sponge sticks, flossers with long handles, electric toothbrushes with rotary brushes (can be held vertically in front of the mouth instead of horizontally at the side))
Portable suction machines
Portable speech synthesizer and word-processing software
   portable hand-held communication device (Crestalk, Crespeak)
   portable personal computers (Lightwriter, Likon), with scanning switches or mouse if hands or fingers cannot manage the keys
   Speak Easy software program for lap-top computers

everything is fine. However, as the disease progresses, new relationships between the patient and caregiver inevitably develop. Family members or friends may drift away, either intentionally or unintentionally. In these situations, the social worker can be instrumental in providing support and reinforcing coping mechanisms.

Support can be provided by one-on-one counseling, family counseling, or support group meetings. For some, meeting and talking with other patients in the clinic is adequate; for others, a support group is beneficial. Such groups are especially helpful for those who, due to restrictions imposed by some healthcare delivery systems, are not able to seek out a specialty clinic setting. In many instances, a portion of the support group meeting is devoted to a lecture or presentation regarding a specific topic. The remaining time is used for open discussion. Patients and caregivers can learn, share ideas and draw support from others who are living with the same disease or caring for someone with ALS. Conversely, there are just as many patients and caregivers who want no part of a support group. The reason cited most often is not wanting to be confronted with seeing others who have the disease. For these, the one-on-one approach is best.

Also, there are people who choose not to gather information from either clinic or support groups but rely on the Internet alone. For those families who live in rural areas where access to either a health care facility or support group is limited, the Internet is a useful source of information and support. However, as healthcare professionals we must caution our patients about 'information' via the Internet; some 'information' is easily misconstrued, inaccurate, or does not actually inform. Patients should be referred to websites run by professional organizations and advocacy groups (see Resources, page 147).

In counseling patients and caregivers, the social worker determines whether or not they should be seen separately. Both patients and caregivers need to be able to freely discuss feelings of anger, resentment, guilt, frustration, loss, fear, death, loneliness and self-doubt.

In addition to tending to the emotional needs of patients, a social worker can be an invaluable resource for community referrals. ALS not only takes a toll physically, but in its later stages can be a terribly expensive disease. In the United States, the social worker must be knowledgeable about financial assistance programs that are available through national or local governmental agencies such as Medicare, Medicaid, Social Security Disability, Veterans Administration and Supplemental Security Income (SSI) or life insurance viaticals.

Viatical settlements are a new death benefit of life insurance whereby insurance funds are signed over to a settlement provider before the death of the insured. In return, the provider gives the terminally ill patient a percentage of the worth of the policy based on the diagnosis and prognosis of the illness. The patient and family then have money to provide care for the patient until death. If patients are not eligible for such programs, they must use their own financial resources, which can quickly dwindle in order to purchase expensive equipment, home care, medications and treatment options.

In Europe, each country has its own system of national and private healthcare, with or without additional private health insurance coverage and life insurance provisions. Long-term ventilation is typically not an option. However, in the United States, Canada, and Japan, patients are often given a choice to receive mechanical ventilation for respiratory insufficiency.

As the physical challenge of caring for a loved one mounts, the caretaker's role becomes more demanding. The focus may switch to the caregiver's health and well-being. Based on financial status and insurance coverage, a number of options are available which the social worker helps explore. In most cases, patients with ALS will be cared for at home instead of a facility such as a nursing home. Recommendations about the use of private nursing agencies, governmental assistive programs, community programs, respite programs and hospices must be explored to assist in the physical care aspects. Recruitment efforts through church groups and nursing school students can provide much needed part-time relief. In addition, some communities have placement programs which provide 24 hour live-in care in exchange for room and board and a small salary.

It must be acknowledged that patients and their families will undergo numerous adjustments in coping with ALS. We recognize their fears and concerns and treat the depression which is a very real component of this disease. Mobilizing patients to draw upon their strengths and encouraging them to participate in enjoyable life activities fosters an attitude of realistic hope.

Physical therapist's role

Most ALS patients seek to maintain mobility and ambulation as long as possible. To achieve these goals, the PT provides instruction in maintaining muscle strength and joint mobility, preventing joint stiffness and pain, slowing muscle atrophy, facilitating ambulation, and demonstrating proper body mechanics, thereby preventing injury and muscle strain to both the patient and caregiver.

Maintaining mobility of the upper and lower extremities requires a simple daily regimen of range-of-motion exercises before rising from bed in the morning and before falling asleep at night. These can be active, active-assistive or passive exercises. Shoulder flexion and rotations can be performed while lying on the bed with or without pillow support. These exercises must be initiated early to maintain joint mobility and prevent 'frozen shoulders'. When carried out in the early and later stages, they help prevent joint and muscle stiffness and pain and permit easier dressing, bathing and hygiene by the patient or caregiver. Combined isometric contraction of ankle dorsiflexors, knee extensors and hip flexors can be performed while lying in bed or sitting in a chair to maintain strength in the lower extremities. This simple exercise is performed periodically during the day by alternating legs and holding the contraction for 6 seconds. Isometric exercise involves the contraction and relaxation of muscle without the actual movement of limbs. The weight of the limbs alone is usually sufficient for a general exercise program. Depending on the degree of weakness, using 5 or 10 lb (2–5 kg) weights may cause muscle fatigue, muscle strain in the wrist, hand, shoulder or low back areas. Exercises can be limited to short, periodic sets if excessive muscle fatigue is a problem. Patients should be reminded that rest is needed following exercise for muscle strength recuperation. A home program of exercises that a patient can perform daily will be of benefit to both patient and caregiver. Periodic assessment of muscle strength re-emphasizes the importance of performing exercises.

Patients need to walk as much as possible, whether at home or at work. Sitting in one place for more than one hour should be discouraged, because stiffness and weakness increase with immobility. Need for assistive devices such as canes, ankle-foot orthoses, walkers and seat-lift recliner chairs must be presented as positive aids to continued independence. Even patients whose mobility is limited by muscle weakness and poor respiratory endurance should be encouraged to stand every hour with support and practice walking in place or shifting balance from one side to the other. This maintains hip flexion and extension, knee extension, neck and trunk extension and coordination.

Simple breathing exercises that encourage increased inspiration, expiration, expansion of the chest cavity and excursion of the diaphragm should be initiated early. Short, repetitive exercises that can be performed periodically during the day without devices will give the patient opportunity to concentrate on this activity without fatiguing respiratory muscles.

Pulmonologist's role

Depending on the experience of the principal ALS physician, patients are sometimes referred to a pulmonologist when respiratory function is compromised and assistive ventilation options are considered. Since respiratory failure is the main cause of death in ALS patients, the physician should assess vital capacity at all clinic visits to monitor the disease progression. The proper timing for discussions about pulmonary assistance, gastrostomy placement, quality of life, hospice, advanced directives and end-of-life care depends on measurement of respiratory function. This is usually done when the forced vital capacity declines to about 50% of predicted. Measurement of slow or forced vital capacity and inspiratory/expiratory volumes can be done formally in the pulmonary function lab or during an outpatient clinic visit with a hand-held spirometer. Breathing exercises and proper positioning for eating and sleeping can improve respiratory excursion and prevent discomfort.

The physician should explore the patient's knowledge and wishes for long-term or end-of-life measures. Elective tracheostomy and the use of BiPAP, CPAP, or supplemental oxygen as 'bridges' to a ventilator or as comfort care can be thoroughly explained and considered. When not the principal care physician, the pulmonologist should still assist with quality-of-life decisions which may or may not have been discussed during clinic or office visits. Tables 7.6 and 7.7 list recommendations for improved breathing techniques and assistive devices.

Because of its complexity, long-term care at home must be planned for by the physician, patient, family members and medical team professionals. Desire by the patient to continue living with life support involves:

1 Sufficient financial resources to support this decision, whether it is in the form of insurance coverage, public assistance or personal resources to pay for 24-hour care.
2 Physical ability and willingness of family members to support this decision and actually take on some of the daily care of the patient.
3 Clear, written advance directives for continuation or cessation of life support if conditions change. Such changes may be medical, financial, and personal or family issues.

Hospice care is a most valuable option for those who do not choose long-term life support. Patients and families benefit from the hospice orientation to

Table 7.6 Recommendations for improved breathing

Pursed lip/diaphragmatic breathing exercises done periodically during each day encourage chest
  expansion and controlled breathing to improve volume and reduce anxiety
Small, frequent meals decrease abdominal pressure, and allow diaphragm to work more efficiently
Partially reclined position in bed allows diaphragmatic movement
Sitting or partially reclined position after meals allow proper digestion and reduce pressure against
  the diaphragm

Table 7.7 Respiratory assistive devices

Portable suction machine with Yankauer catheters
Intermittent positive pressure breathing (IPPB) device – small respirator used for occasional breathing
  problems; should be humidified
CPAP: continuous positive assistive pressure, used with a nasal mask to rest breathing muscles up to
  24 hours
BiPAP: inspiratory and expiratory pressures set to assist breathing, used with a nasal mask or nasal
  pillows
Tracheostomy: procedure to open the airway, provides for easier suctioning of throat secretions,
  usually needs ventilatory assistance
Positive pressure ventilation: part or full-time mechanical ventilatory assistance, used when
  non-invasive ventilation does not provide sufficient support, or patient cannot tolerate nasal
  mask/pillows.

provide comfort services in the form of dressing or bathing aides, medical equipment, medication to prevent discomfort or anxiety, and regular or immediate medical services at home.

Speech therapist's role

The speech therapist assesses the patient's ability to communicate and swallow. Speech and swallowing muscles include the lips, tongue, palate, larynx and respiratory muscles. Spasticity and weakness of these areas cause imprecise articulation, hypernasality, hoarseness, monotone speech, reduced volume in speech, and choking or aspiration when swallowing.

Techniques for improved speech are provided. These include using a slower, overarticulated speech, substituting words that are easier to pronounce, using exaggerated pitch or loudness, and regulating breathing before talking. The listener should follow some simple rules: eliminate noise and other distractions; face the patient and concentrate on listening; allow the patient to speak for him- or herself; tell the patient when you do not understand; encourage short phrases or substitution of simpler words. Recommendations for alternate communication techniques and electronic speech synthesizer devices are presented in Table 7.8.

The speech therapist performs periodic oral pharyngeal motility or swallow tests to record deglutition and any apparent aspiration. Recommended swallowing techniques include positioning the chin downward after the bolus of food has been moved to the back of the oral cavity and elimination of distractions. Recommendations for change in food and liquid consistencies, specific chewing, swallowing and cough techniques, or suggestions about alternative feeding methods (gastrostomy or percutaneous endoscopic gastrostomy) are made.

Table 7.8 Communication devices

Voice/telephone amplifier if dysarthria is not present
Communication boards (alphabet, E-Tran)
Portable electronic communication devices which are hand-held with keyboard activation (Crestalk, Crespeaker, Canon communicator, Link, Lightwriter)
Head pointer, light pointer (attached to headband) or mouth stick
Electronic switches (touch, eyebrow, eyeblink switches, scanning device) used to activate computer keyboard
Adapted telephones, speaker phones with speed dial, operator headrest and phone holders
Telephone services relay messages: TTY/TDD (Telecommunication device for the deaf)
Computers with hardware, software and modem, modified with electronic switches or voice activated programs to conduct business transactions and communicate electronically (e-mail)

Assisted cough techniques, which include a 'huffing' squeeze cough and 'frog breathing', can be demonstrated, and recommendations made for use of a cough machine or in-exsufflator.

Nutritionist's role

Good nutrition provides a source of energy, helps maintain muscle, prevents weight loss, and may strengthen the immune system. However, maintaining good nutrition for the ALS patient is easier said than done. One of the inevitable effects of ALS is bulbar involvement. As bulbar muscles become weaker, patients experience increased difficulty in eating. Initially, they will deny swallowing problems, and questions need to be framed around specifics such as choking, length of time it takes to eat, weight loss, and elimination of various foods such as crackers or popcorn. As time passes, it becomes increasingly difficult to swallow food of any consistency, and the once enjoyable act of eating becomes a chore. A vicious cycle develops when the patient knows he or she should eat but quickly fatigues and loses the desire to continue eating. The time and energy required to eat a meal may be more than patients can handle. Couple this with a caregiver's concern that the loved one is not eating and losing weight, and a mealtime can become an anxious ordeal.

In order to help patients maintain good nutrition, periodic assessment of their nutritional status is needed as the disease progresses. This means recommending ways of increasing caloric and protein consumption, suggesting changes in food consistency, and guiding the choice of nutritional supplements (see Table 7.9). In some clinic settings, a nutritionist is available to assist with an evaluation of caloric and nutritional needs. However, if one is not available, the patient's nutritional needs must still be assessed. Patients should be weighed at each clinic visit so that weight loss can be identified and appropriate recommendations made about diet supplementation. It may be advisable to undertake a swallowing imaging study to further assess a patient's ability to swallow. However, severity on cine-esophagram or video fluoroscopy generally precedes severity as judged by the patient. Based on the results, recommendations can be weighed concerning dietary changes. This can involve either changes in food consistency, or (if aspiration is noted) alternate feeding methods.

Obviously, we want our patients to maintain their caloric intake in a manner they can easily tolerate. One of the first recommendations that should be

Table 7.9 Increasing caloric intake

Nutritional drinks (e.g., Ensure, Sustacal, Carnation Instant Breakfast)
Fruit juice
Milk with chocolate syrup
Use of sauces, gravy, jam, jelly, sugar
Addition of extra fat (butter, margarine, cream) to mashed potatoes, hot cereals, soups, noodles, vegetables
Dairy products – pudding, fruited yogurt, ice-cream, cheese, milkshakes, whipped cream
Pancakes, waffles with syrup
Candy bars
Substitute soy products if milk causes increased phlegm

made is to eat five to six small meals a day instead of the usual three. The anxiety, frustration and fatigue factor that often accompanies the act of eating can therefore be alleviated. Well-balanced meals and modified food preparation are recommended. Commercially prepared supplements that provide 250–350 calories per serving increase caloric intake. Some patients cannot tolerate canned supplements but are able to substitute powdered breakfast drinks prepared with whole milk instead. Special cookbooks, especially *Meals for Easy Swallowing* from the Muscular Dystrophy Association, are particularly useful for providing palatable recipes that will provide the necessary calories, protein and nutrients.

When patients can no longer adequately or safely meet nutritional needs and the risk of aspiration is identified, feeding tubes should be considered. A thorough discussion with the patient and caregiver must take place to weigh all options, including potential risks and complications. It is advisable to introduce the topic of a feeding tube when patients first begin to experience dysphagia. They need time to determine whether or not a feeding tube is in their best interest. Despite stereotypes, a feeding tube does not necessarily represent an 'extraordinary means' or 'heroic measure'. Instead, it is, in a sense, a comfort measure. Less anxiety, more energy, hydration, and adequate nutrition are the positive benefits of a feeding tube. In having this discussion early, the risks involved can potentially be lessened if a tube is inserted before the patient's nutritional or respiratory status are significantly compromised. It must also be noted that having a feeding tube does not necessarily represent the sole means for receiving nutritional support. For many, eating is viewed as a social event. However, when dysphagia becomes severe, patients rarely view mealtime as a pleasant or sociable event. By alleviating the stress and anxiety that often accompany eating, a gastrostomy can save energy to be used for other activities.

A number of procedures are available. In most circumstances, a percutaneous endoscopic gastrostomy (PEG) is used. It is a surgical procedure that allows the patient to be awake while receiving a mild sedative, thereby lessening the potential for postoperative complications. The procedure utilizes endoscopic guidance as a catheter is inserted percutaneously into the stomach. Placement of this type of tube allows for bolus feedings which can be given on a schedule that coincides with normal eating times. An alternate procedure is a gastrojejunostomy. This method is not as convenient as a PEG, especially for the patient who is ambulatory. This catheter is inserted in the jejunum, and, because of its small capacity, bolus feedings are not always feasible. Nutritional supplementation is delivered via a kangaroo pump and given over a 10–12 hour period. Therefore, it is recommended that feedings be delivered during the evening hours. Although this is an acceptable alternative to a PEG, the patient who is mobile will find this a very restrictive means of receiving nutritional support. The least desirable option for long-term nutritional management is the nasogastric tube. Complications such as nasopharyngeal discomfort, irritation, aspiration and dislodgement can occur.

Conclusion

The multidisciplinary team approach has developed into a comprehensive system for the management and support of ALS patients. Assessment and symptomatic treatment by each discipline is aimed at improving physical and emotional well-being, as well as the quality of lives.

Acknowledgements

We are grateful to the ALS patients and families who have taught us how to care for them most effectively these past 20 years. We have also been privileged to work with other dedicated health professionals in our respective clinics. Special thanks go to Amy Casey for her editing assistance and to Drs Irwin Siegel and Robert Sufit for their medical advice.

Suggested reading

Miller R et al. (1997) Amyotrophic Lateral Sclerosis Standard of Care Consensus Conference. Neurology 48 (Suppl 4):S1–S37.

Caroscio JT (1986) Amyotrophic Lateral Sclerosis: A Guide to Patient Care. Thieme Medical Publishers Inc: New York.

Mitsumoto H, Munsat T (2001) Amyotrophic Lateral Sclerosis: A Guide for Patients and Families, 2nd Edition. Demos Medical Publishing Inc.: New York.

Resources

The following is a list of organizations that are wonderful resources for patients and caregivers.

The Amyotrophic Lateral Sclerosis Association (ALSA)

27001 Agoura Rd., Suite 150
Calabasas Hills, CA 91301–5104 USA
Tel.:   +1 (818) 880-9007
Fax: +1 (818) 880-9006
Patient hotline: +1 (800) 782-4747
Website: http://www.alsa.org

Muscular Dystrophy Association (MDA)

3300 E. Sunrise Drive
Tucson, AZ 85718
Tel.:   +1 (602) 529 2000
Fax: +1 (602) 529 5300
Patient Information: +1 (800) 572 1717
Website: http://www.mdausa.org

Motor Neuron Disease Association

P.O. Box 246
Northampton, NNI 2PR, UK
Tel.:   +44 1604 250505
Fax: +44 1604 638289
Website: http://www.mndassociation.org

Amyotrophic Lateral Sclerosis Society of Canada

6 Adelaide Street East, Suite 220
Toronto, Ontario M5C 1H6
Tel.:   +1 (416) 362 0269
Fax: +1 (416) 362 0414
Outside Toronto: +1 (800) 276 4257
Website: http://www.als.ca/alssociety.shtml

Therapeutic trials, drug development, and regulatory oversight

Frank Baldino Jr, John M. Farah Jr, and Ralph W. Kuncl

Introduction

In this chapter, we attempt to associate selected elements that have emerged from clinical and basic research related to the motor unit which are important, in our view, to the design and interpretation of clinical investigations in patients with motor neuron disease (MND, amyotrophic lateral sclerosis). Although this discussion considers several of the major developments in the field, it is not meant to be a comprehensive review, as it draws heavily from Cephalon's experience with the development of recombinant human insulin like growth factor-1 (rhIGF-1) for MND. Parallels are also drawn between progress made in clinical research and a changing regulatory environment. The last 10 years has witnessed tremendous advances in our understanding of the clinical course of MND (see Chapter 1) as well as the cellular and molecular mechanisms at the core of its etiology (discussed in Chapter 3).

New research tools for drug development

Considerable emphasis during this period has been placed on elucidating some of the fundamental cellular mechanisms of motor neuron death, axonal regeneration, and axonal sprouting. Several laboratories have identified a host of factors which may either mediate or impinge on the process of neuronal loss. These studies have implicated several molecules, reviewed in some detail in Chapter 3, including glutamate, calcium, autoantibodies, neurotrophic factors, the caspases, the Bcl family of cell death modulators, and several reactive oxygen species, as possibly contributing to the process of motor neuron death. Also in the past decade, a genetic link was identified in a population of patients suffering from a familial form of this disease (Rosen et al., 1993). The identity of a number of specific mutations in the nucleic acid sequence coding for Cu/Zn superoxide dismutase provided important insights into the genetic nature of familial MND. This important link has spawned considerable interest for others to expand upon that initial discovery and has resulted in the development of a number of transgenic animal models of familial MND (Gurney et al., 1994, 1996) and superoxide dismutase (SOD) knockouts (Reaume et al., 1996) to study the role of the enzyme and oxidative stress in MND (see Chapters 4 and 6). These advances have provided scientists with long-awaited research tools to further advance our understanding of the mechanisms of motor neuron death and the extent to which the regeneration and sprouting properties of axons compensate for the loss of motor neurons.

Lessons from recent therapeutic trials

The 1990s witnessed an unprecedented level of pharmaceutical investment in clinical trials, with no fewer than 12 corporate products entering clinical development for MND since 1993, including riluzole (Bensimon et al., 1994; Lacomblez et al., 1996), recombinant growth hormone (Smith et al., 1993), recombinant human ciliary neurotrophic factor (rhCNTF) (ALS CNTF Treatment Study Phase II-III Study Group, 1996; Miller et al., 1996d), nimodipine (Miller et al., 1996b), gabapentin (Miller et al., 1996a; Mazzini et al., 1998; Scrip Daily Online, Nov 1999), rhIGF-1 (Myotrophin® [mecasermin] Injection) (Lai et al., 1997), superoxide dismutase (Cudkowicz et al., 1997), xaliproden (Mucke and Castañer, 1998), recombinant human brain derived neurotrophic factor (rhBDNF) (BDNF Study Group, 1999; Cedarbaum et al., 2000), recombinant human glial cell-line derived neurotrophic factor (rhGDNF) (Bohn, 1999), LY300164, and topiramate. To date riluzole, rhIGF-1, rhBDNF, and xaliproden have shown intriguing results in clinical trials, but only riluzole and rhIGF-1 have been approved or received an approvable status for commercialization. These regulatory decisions were based on the demonstration that riluzole increases patient survival and rhIGF-1 slows disease progression and sustains quality of life. The initial trials of xaliproden missed statistical significance.

The putative mechanisms of action for both rhIGF-1 and riluzole are compelling. They represent an extraordinary example in neurology of how the effects of a molecule in preclinical laboratory studies can predict a clinical effect in humans. Among the documented actions of riluzole include its ability to prevent the release of glutamate and to partially antagonize the NMDA class of excitatory amino acid receptor. There is a rich literature detailing the role of excitatory amino acids (EAA) in inducing neuronal death (Shaw and Ince, 1997). This EAA hypothesis was extended to motor neurons and MND by discoveries from the Kuncl and Rothstein laboratories indicating elevated spinal fluid glutamate and aspartate (Rothstein et al., 1991), a defective glutamate transporter in spinal cord and motor cortex (Rothstein et al., 1992, 1995), and the ability to model specific motor neuron damage experimentally by inhibition of the glutamate transporter (Rothstein et al., 1993, 1996). Thus, the preclinical and clinical effects of riluzole attest to the plausibility of excitotoxicity in the pathogenesis of MND.

Recombinant human IGF-1 is unique in that this pleiotrophic protein positively influences each component of the motor unit. All of the effects of rhIGF-1 are mediated by a specific high affinity receptor which has been localized to lower motor neurons and motor nerve terminals at the neuromuscular junction (Lewis et al., 1993). Research over the past 10 years has demonstrated that IGF-1 is a potent neurotrophic factor with a significant effect on inhibiting the process of cellular apoptosis in several types of neurons, including motor neurons. It has been shown to be neurotrophic or neuroprotective for motor neurons in the face of several experimental challenges, including excitotoxicity (Corse et al., 1999), axotomy (Contreras et al., 1995), and Fe^{2+}-induced oxidative damage (Doré et al., 1997).

In addition to its role in preventing apoptosis, the neurotrophic actions of IGF-1 extend to peripheral nerve regeneration and sprouting where it has been clearly demonstrated to mediate axonal regeneration (Hansson et al., 1985) and both nodal and junctional sprouting (Caroni and Grandes, 1990). The ability of rhIGF-1 to slow the progression of disease in patients with MND and maintain a higher quality of life (Lai et al., 1997) suggests an even broader therapeutic rationale for neurotrophism in neurodegenerative disease.

At the very least, these studies demonstrate that both riluzole and rhIGF-1 are active in patients with a neurodegenerative disease. These demonstrations in clinical trials provide the neurology community with important tools that have not previously been available, the lack of which has severely limited advances in the field.

Issues in drug development

Amyotrophic lateral sclerosis (ALS) has been designated by the Food and Drug Administration (FDA) as an orphan disease because its prevalence in the US population is less than 210 000. It is remarkable, therefore, that an orphan indication such as ALS would garner such significant corporate investments when the rate of financial returns are not likely to justify the cost of drug development. This is particularly the case considering 1990s biomedical technology and the present regulatory environment.

Nevertheless, several new products have entered the development cycle and completed clinical trials. Is it a desire for innovation, a quest for new knowledge, or simply altruism that belies this relatively recent behavior in large and small pharmaceutical companies? Although these are clearly motivating factors for any scientist, MND has become a surrogate to test a principle which is critical to future progress in neurology. It is an approach to answer the seminal question of whether or not we can positively impact the progression of any neurodegenerative disease.

Several characteristics of MND render this disorder a compelling form of neurodegenerative disease for clinical study. Primary among these is that although MND is a neuronal disease, it can be studied with outcome measures designed to evaluate muscle function. These outcome measures allow for facile quantification, more so than many of the neurological outcomes that are currently available in other disorders. In addition, the compromised population of neurons (in this example, the lower motor neurons), although residing within the central nervous system compartment, extend beyond the blood–brain barrier into the peripheral nervous system. Thus, the axons and terminals of these neurons are convenient and accessible targets for a wider range of potential therapeutic agents for which blood–brain barrier permeability would normally be a limitation.

Another attractive feature of MND for clinical study, although devastating to patients and their families, is the rapid rate of progression of this disease. This precipitous decline allows not only for a reasonable time course of study which spans a significant portion of the natural progression of disease, but also for the correlation of muscle dysfunction, and potentially neuronal death, with the survival of the patient. This correlation is an opportunity that is difficult to achieve with other neurodegenerative conditions that progress at a far more indolent pace.

The ability of the international neurological community to conduct successful placebo controlled multicenter trials demonstrates that therapeutic agents can be developed that impact this disease. In particular, the results of the riluzole and rhIGF-1 studies demonstrate a clinically meaningful retardation of disease progression. These findings, for the first time, suggest that the once unachievable goal of slowing the progression of a chronic neurodegenerative disease *can* be accomplished.

Difficulties in trial design from the point of view of the pharmaceutical industry

Certainly the inability to conduct small focused studies in MND has seriously hampered drug development efforts. There have been few examples of success in MND clinical studies of any size, but especially in studies that randomize fewer than 300 patients (rhIGF-1 studies randomized 455 patients in two separate studies). A successful trial in a small study population would permit more insightful and sensible designs of pivotal phase III studies and mitigate a portion of the risk associated with conducting large and expensive trials to achieve a first approximation of a drug effect. Even the failed clinical studies in MND have provided valuable insights into aspects of this disease. For example, the failure of rhCNTF underscored the need to fully develop the pharmacokinetic safety profile of any new agent before any clinical evaluation of efficacy. Similarly, the promising results of rhBDNF in a Phase II study and its subsequent failure in a larger Phase III study focused the field on the importance of responsive subgroups, the risk of prolonged study duration, and the high degree of variability associated with the use of forced vital capacity as an endpoint in an MND clinical trial. Furthermore, these experiences have defined several important variables and prognostic factors that exert a profound influence on the interpretation of well controlled clinical investigations, as well as design of future studies.

Heterogeneity and stratification

The heterogeneity of MND patients stands out as the most influential variable within trial results that hampers the interpretation of these studies. For example, patients with predominately bulbar disease or bulbar-onset disease usually differ in their clinical course and generally survive for a shorter period of time than limb-onset patients. In addition, there are important differences between upper and lower limb onset that need to be accounted for in a proper clinical study. For small focused clinical studies, imbalances between treatment groups in the type of disease at onset may preclude a valid interpretation of the results because the fundamental requirement for statistical comparisons between 'like' groups would have been violated. For example, studies that are meant to probe for preliminary evidence of clinical effect may be designed to enroll only patients with rapidly progressing disease or with bulbar onset disease. While the enrollment of such a study may be lengthy due to the more stringent inclusion and exclusion criteria, the actual treatment phase of such a study may be considerably shorter than one in which a broad range of patients with MND are eligible. More important than the cost of conducting such a study is that interpretable evidence of drug effect is more likely to be detectable in the narrow, homogeneous patient population and the results of such a study may become available sooner than in an exploratory study in a broad spectrum of patients with MND. Such outcomes are desirable in the industry from the perspective of critical go/no go decisions in a drug candidate's 'life cycle' as well as for the design and conduct of pivotal clinical trials. The limitation, of course, is the less broad applicability of the study's outcome.

Stratification of patients between treatment groups and clinical centers as to the form of their disease is crucial to address the issue of heterogeneity among MND patients and to preserve proper comparability of treatment groups. Randomization of patients with different forms of disease becomes less of an issue in larger studies of greater than 1000 patients where adequate randomization may occur by chance alone.

Outcome measures

The choice of outcome measures in these clinical studies has also been controversial. The desire for quantification has to be balanced with the demands by the neurology community and national regulatory agencies for clinical relevance. Demonstration of a quantitative slowing in the deterioration of muscle strength in a particular type of muscle needs to be coupled with the impact on an MND patient's clinical condition, and ultimately, quality of life. The clinical importance of a 15% slowing of muscle dysfunction in the tibialis anterior muscle, as an example, may not be apparent to all neurologists and federal regulators even if it is statistically highly significant. Quantitative assessments of muscle function in isolated muscle groups would also complicate trial design because the comparison of treatment effects in isolated muscle groups between patients may be greatly affected by the type of disease at onset and variability in the extent of the loss of motor neurons in the selected muscle group. Nevertheless, such objective measures of a potential drug effect on biological function can be quite compelling considerations to justify the approval of a new drug application.

Several neuromuscular centers have developed ordinal clinimetric scales over the years which attempt to combine a degree of quantification of muscle function with important assessments of clinical relevance. These scales span the broad range between quantitative and qualitative clinical assessments. For example, the Norris scale (Norris et al., 1974; Brooks, 1994) provides important clinical data with little quantitative information, whereas the TQNE (Tufts Quantitative Neuromuscular Exam; Andres et al., 1986) provides important quantitative data with less clinical information. The Appel ALS scale (AALS) (Appel et al., 1987) may balance the two extremes at the expense of mixing subjective and quantitative assessments that evaluate elements of disease disabilities and handicaps. Finally, the ALS Functional Rating Scale (ALS CNTF Treatment Study [ACTS] Phase I–II Study Group, 1996) is a simple, patient-based subjective questionnaire which focuses on the disability of MND. What is clear from clinical investigations to date is that while none of these ordinal scales is a perfect clinical instrument, each independently corroborates the clinical and patient-based perspective on the chronic, relentless course of MND (Brooks, 1996).

The selection of a clinical endpoint is not without consequence from a regulatory perspective. For example, the selection of survival provides distinct regulatory advantages in the USA in that specific regulations exist which effectively lower the requirements for approval if survival is a prospectively defined endpoint and a drug candidate demonstrates a statistically significant survival advantage. On the other hand, leading clinical authorities and patient advocates have questioned the value of a product that promotes survival of MND patients without a positive impact on the deterioration of muscle function and a patient's quality of life. Since an important component of regulatory approval in the USA is concurrence by a panel of medical experts as to the clinical relevance of any new therapy, these two perspectives appear to be at odds with one another. This important issue remains unsettled in the field. The apparent conflict will be resolved when MND therapies are created which offer patients both extended lifespan and sustained quality of life.

The selection among ordinal scales is also not without consequence, as the general acceptance of each of these clinical instruments varies among clinicians and institutions. Ironically, the persistence of this point of view is difficult to comprehend in the face of data that demonstrates the remarkable correlation between each of these validated scales. This particular issue is of lesser relevance from a regulatory perspective, where any validated and clinically relevant scale can be used to support the approval of a product. Whatever the choice of ordinal scale, the rate of change of disease as assessed by each scale is highly correlated with survival (Preux et al., 1996). For example, the AALS rating scale has been used in characterizing the natural history of patients with MND. Patients who progress rapidly display a higher relative risk of early death than those progressing at a less aggressive pace (Haverkamp et al., 1995). Using the median rate of progression for all patients enrolled in the North American trial of IGF-1 to demarcate 'rapid' and 'slow' progressors, (i.e. 4 AALS points per month, as applied to the natural history database of nearly 1500 patients from Baylor University), it becomes evident that patients with MND progressing rapidly are at significantly greater risk of death than patients progressing more slowly (Figure 8.1).

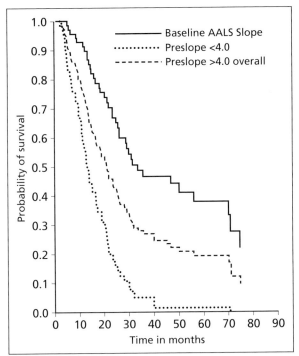

Fig. 8.1 Kaplan–Meier survival curves for Baylor database. A database of patients with MND who were followed at Baylor College of Medicine (Haverkamp et al., 1995) was queried for those patients who would have met the criteria for randomization to the North American study of rhIGF-1. Of all patients in the database at the time of the query, there were 141 who would have passed the inclusion and exclusion criteria for the study and for whom a pre-randomization slope in the AALS scoring system was evaluable. Of those 141 eligible patients, 71 who demonstrated a preslope rate of decline equal to or less than 4 AALS points per month (slow progressors) were at a far lower risk of death than those 70 patients who demonstrated a preslope rate of decline greater than 4 AALS points per month (fast progressors)

Prognostic factors

Notwithstanding this simple observation, both the dependent and independent cascade of this simple correlation are profoundly influenced by at least three important prognostic factors: age, forced vital capacity (FVC), and site of disease onset (Preux et al., 1996; Louwerse et al., 1996, 1997). The influence of age as prognostic for survival is easily understood and firmly established in the literature (Preux et al., 1996; Louwerse et al., 1997). Patients who are diagnosed with MND at an older age are at significantly higher risk of death than those diagnosed younger. The interactions of FVC, clinical form of disease, and disease progression present a more complicated picture.

Disease progression

The need to fully consider this important interrelationship in the design of a relatively small focused clinical trial in MND can be better understood using data from the rhIGF-1 studies. Consider two patients, one a limb-onset patient with progressing disease in the lumbar cord, the other a bulbar-onset patient with progressing disease in the cervical cord. Let's assume that both patients have similar baseline AALS scores and are rapid progressors, each progressing at 6.0 AALS points per month. On the basis of published data, the bulbar-onset patient would be expected to die within 1–2 years of diagnosis as a result of respiratory failure, while the limb-onset patient would be expected to die approximately 3–4 years from diagnosis, also from respiratory failure, despite having an identical rate of disease progression (Louwerse et al., 1997). In the rhIGF-1 studies, the median survival times for placebo-treated patients, using Kaplan–Meier methods, were 586 days in the European study and 517 days in the North American study. Patients with bulbar involvement had respective median survival times of 383 and 348 days. Consistent with previous studies, patients in these trials with bulbar onset survived for a dramatically shorter period of time than patients with limb onset of MND (Table 8.1).

Site of onset

This example illustrates two concepts that are important in trial design and interpretation. One is that the survival of MND patients differs markedly depending on the clinical form of disease at presentation. The other is that, although *within* each clinical form of MND there is a clear correlation between rate of progression of disease (rate of decline in muscle dysfunction) and survival, *between* the clinical forms at onset there are dramatic differences in progression of disease and survival (Preux et al., 1996; Louwerse et al., 1997).

Notwithstanding the loss of upper motor neurons, the pathophysiology of MND may be viewed as a contiguous loss of motor neurons within the longitudinal axis of the spinal cord. Typically, lumbar-onset disease progresses rostrally affecting, in temporal sequence, the lower limbs, upper limbs, and eventually the bulbar and respiratory musculature (Brooks, 1996). There have been exceedingly few instances of lower limb-onset disease being immediately followed by significant respiratory impairment. Conversely, motor neuron loss in bulbar-onset patients proceeds caudally to the upper and then lower limbs. Bulbar-onset patients may take years to develop lower limb symptoms and may

Table 8.1 Median survival for North American and European pivotal studies of rhIGF-1 in patients with MND

	Median survival (days)	
	North America	Europe
Overall	517	586
Bulbar onset	348	383
Other onset*	615	623

*Upper or lower limb onset or combination thereof.

die before any significant lower limb involvement (Brooks, 1996), thus affecting fewer elements of global clinimetric scales like the AALS. As a consequence, the total severity of MND at end stage disease will be scored lower among bulbar-onset patients on average than lower limb-onset MND patients. In the latter patient, loss of lower limb function is usually followed by upper limb then bulbar (including respiratory) involvement (Brooks, 1996). Thus, in contrast to the course of a bulbar-onset patient, the muscle deterioration in these patients involves most, if not all, of the components of a global clinimetric scale, driving, for example, the total AALS score at death in some cases near its maximum of 160 points. Upper limb patients are the most unpredictable in this regard, and consequently the most variable population in their clinical course. Their disease may progress rostrally or caudally within the cord. Rostral progression in an upper limb patient will result in a relatively shorter survival time and a lower AALS score than caudal progression (Brooks, 1996). Consequently, the global clinimetric scores achieved by bulbar and limb onset patients differ markedly and may appear to correlate less well with survival (Haverkamp et al., 1995) than groups stratified on the basis of time since disease onset.

No one understands what determines the site of disease onset in MND. However, it is clear that patients usually do not die from generalized muscle dysfunction but rather from dysfunction of the musculature involved in respiration. Hence, unless euthanasia or fatal intercurrent illnesses are involved, essentially all MND patients die from respiratory failure. Although there is a correlation between chronic muscle deterioration and survival, this correlation is only clearly evident within each clinical form (i.e. bulbar, upper limb, or lower limb patients) of disease (Preux et al., 1996; Louwerse et al., 1997). For a clinical trial in which randomization was successful (i.e. resulted in a balanced representation of each of the three clinical forms of disease across treatment groups) there should be an excellent correlation between progression of disease and survival, with significantly less variance within strata defined by site of onset.

Respiratory status

FVC may be a valuable normalizer among MND patients due to the ultimate hazard of respiratory failure. It should be no surprise that FVC is highly correlated with survival (Louwerse et al., 1996): patients who breathe well at baseline, as demonstrated by a favorable FVC, will generally fare better in the course of a clinical trial than those who demonstrate impaired respiratory capacity at baseline. Although FVC at baseline is positively correlated with duration of survival, survival in patients with similar FVCs is also very much influenced by the clinical form of their disease onset (Preux et al., 1996; Louwerse et al., 1997). A patient with substantial bulbar involvement and a 'good' FVC will survive longer than a bulbar patient with a 'poor' FVC; nonetheless, such a patient will not survive as long, on average, as a lower limb-onset patient with 'good' FVC. One perspective to consider is that disease progression modulates the influence of FVC on survival. Thus, within MND patients grouped by FVC at baseline, there may be a gradient of survival response to treatment based on disease progression. Longer survival is expected in patients with slow disease progression and high FVC at baseline than in patients with lower baseline FVC and rapid disease progression.

Typically, bulbar-onset patients fall into the latter category (Preux et al., 1996). A limitation of the use of FVC as an outcome in clinical trials is the high variance of FVC, due to both technical factors of various measuring devices and the way in which upper motor neuron deficits affect the patient's ability to perform the test. High variance lowers power and requires a larger N.

Taken together, these observations suggest that in parallel group trial design a correlation between treatment effects on survival and muscle deterioration in a population dichotomized by any single factor (e.g. bulbar vs. limb disease) would not be evident unless the treatment groups were also balanced with respect to age, FVC, and type of disease at onset. This would suggest that a clinical trial with a small number of patients may yield interpretable results only if patients were homogeneous with respect to type of MND at onset and stratified for FVC and age.

Surrogate markers

Clinical studies of MND have long been stymied by the lack of surrogate markers for disease activity. The development of clinically important and innovative therapeutic agents for AIDS and cancer have benefitted tremendously from the existence of quantifiable biochemical markers that correlate with substantial elements of disease. Quantitative MRI is just beginning to be explored as an important endpoint in neurology trials and was used in the early 1990s as an independent corroborating result in a trial of recombinant human interferon-1 for multiple sclerosis (Paty et al., 1993). The impact of markedly improved imaging technology for clinical studies in MND is less clear at this time. Nevertheless, MR spectroscopy may be a feasible technology to detect and track pathogenic changes in patients with MND. Recent studies suggest that focused analysis of selected subcortical structures by MR spectroscopy reveals deterioration of neuronal biochemical markers consistent with the losses detected clinically and postmortem. The technology and expertise for MR spectroscopy in MND is not nearly as widespread as the tools for motor unit estimation (discussed below). The potential advantage of MR spectroscopy is that it is not limited to analysis of the lower motor neuron but can assess different populations of neurons affected by disease.

In recent years, several studies have demonstrated some potentially useful electrophysiological outcome measures, such as motor unit number estimation (MUNE), which allows correlation of the estimated number of remaining motor neurons with muscle strength in the evaluable muscle groups innervated by a single peripheral nerve. The results, to date, indicate that motor units are lost at a nonlinear (exponential) rate which belies the apparent monotonic functional loss. This may be explained by compensatory reinnervation of orphaned muscle fibers by surviving motor neurons (Wohlfart, 1957). One of these methodologies was used (Felice 1997) to investigate 21 patients in a longitudinal study and positively correlated the loss of motor units with the loss of muscle strength and a decline in the AALS scale. This technology appears to be validated by multiple reports from centers participating in the clinical study of therapeutic drug candidates, indicating that standard use of MUNE in electromyographic laboratories may be a powerful new approach which is capable of providing a reliable level of quantitative and functional information in an affected muscle group (see Gooch and Harati, 2000). The great advantage is the requirement for a relatively small number of subjects. This would additionally provide an important research opportunity for the cost-effective assessment of new potential therapeutic agents prior to the initiation of more complex and costly phase III pivotal studies that are required for regulatory approval worldwide.

Regulatory environment
Orphan drug laws

In 2000, the regulatory environment in the major pharmaceutical marketplaces (European Union [EU], Japan and the USA) is more favorable toward the approval of new therapeutic agents for lifethreatening diseases than at any time in history. There are several governmental programs and regulations designed specifically to encourage the development of products for orphan indications. Orphan diseases generally are defined on epidemiologic factors. Considering the prevalence criteria established in each commercial territory (see Table 8.2), designated orphan diseases must afflict less than 185 000 patients in the EU, less than 90 000 patients in Japan and less than 210 000 patients in the USA.

In the EU, orphan drug laws are relatively new, but a research and development tax credit under the Orphan Drug Act has provided companies in the USA with a tax credit for monies spent in the development of orphan

Table 8.2 Orphan drug law comparisons

Territory	European Union	Japan	USA
Orphan policy implemented	1999	1993	1983
Prevalence criterion (per 100 000)	< 50*	< 40	< 75
Research and development incentives[†]	YES	YES	YES
Regulatory incentives	YES	YES	YES
Marketing exclusivity	10 years[‡]	7 years	7 years

*Or if life-threatening or severely debilitating with insufficient economic incentive despite a prevalence > 50/100 000.

[†]Incentives are territory specific: In Japan, tax credits of up to 6% of direct R & D costs (less any government subsidy); in the EU protocol assistance is availabe to sponsors from the European Agency for the Evaluation of Medicinal Products (EMEA), financial incentives may be availbable from each member starte of the EU, and registration fees may be subsidized in whole or in part; in the USA, tax credits of up to 50% of direct R & D costs. In Japan, the Drug Organization of the Ministry of Health and Welfare may provide direct grants of up to 50% of R & D expenses for development of an orphan drug candidate. For noncommercial entities in the US, direct grants by Office of Orphan Products Development (FDA) are available which have been sufficient for well controlled phase II studies by clinical investigators.

[‡]In the EU, the Committee for Orphan Medicinal Products, a division of the EMEA, may withdraw market exclusivity at the end of 6 years if an EU member state provides evidence that the epidemiologic or economic criteria for orphan designation are no longer applicable or that unreasonable profit is made by the sponsor of the orphan drug. Furthermore, exclusivity in the EU may be 'derogatable' if the sponsor can no longer supply adequate drug to patients, or another sponsor is able to provide substantially the same product displaying safety, efficacy, or overall clinical benefit superior to the existing orphan drug product. Derogation means that a second sponsor may be licensed to commercialize the same orphan product in the EU to remedy the insufficiencies of the original sponsor's product. Nevertheless, the original sponsor may still enjoy some privileges of exclusivity in that the Committee will not accept a new Market Authorization Application for the same drug for the same orphan indication until the expiry of the original period of exclusivity. (Official Journal of the European Communities, L18/1, 22 January 2000).

products since 1984. Historically, this tax advantage was viewed as being rather limited in scope since the losses resulting from the development of a product could not be carried forward year to year. When one considers that it takes 8–10 years to develop a product from inception to product sales, there was little incentive offered by a one-year tax credit at the end of the development cycle in which tens of millions were spent over the decade of the drug's development. This was especially true for an emerging biopharmaceutical company which is unlikely to generate profits until the product is finally approved. In 1996, the US Orphan Drug Law was amended to permit companies to carry forward research and development losses accrued in the development of a product for an orphan disease. This provision greatly strengthens the value of the research and development tax credit and provides a valuable incentive to develop products for these unmet medical needs.

The Orphan Drug Law additionally provides for a 7-year period of exclusivity within the US marketplace for the manufacture of drugs that are approved for an orphan disease. The intent of this provision is to provide a strong incentive to investigate the potential of any therapeutic product, even those without patent protection, for the treatment of an orphan disease. The establishment of the Orphan Drug Branch of the FDA to oversee these provisions and to provide funding for clinical research in orphan indications is an excellent example of how the interests of the American public and clinical medicine for orphan diseases are properly aligned.

The US Orphan Drug Law has been so successful that the EMEA (European Medicine Evaluation Agency) recently drafted its own version of this law. Although it will be difficult (if not impossible) to negotiate a tax credit across the 15 member states, significant advantages in the form of a period exclusivity in the marketplace and certain reimbursement opportunities will provide powerful incentives to develop products for orphan diseases throughout the European Community. Japan has already adopted an orphan drug provision that expedites the approval process based on the approval of a drug for an orphan disease in another territory.

The US Food and Drug Administration

The US federal standard for the FDA's approval of drugs for commercialization is that a sponsor's clinical studies must provide 'substantial evidence' that a drug is safe and efficacious in treating a disease. The regulations and guidance provided to support that standard apply equally across all FDA divisions, no matter which type of disease or pharmaceutical agent is in a particular division's purview. Nevertheless, there is considerable latitude in the interpretation of these provisions by each division. Although the substantial evidence standard has been traditionally met by two placebo controlled pivotal studies in which the prospectively defined endpoints have reached a statistical threshold of $P < 0.05$, the application of this standard has varied across divisions and clinical indications. For example, in neurology, approval of interferon-1 for multiple sclerosis and of tissue plasminogen activator for stroke was based on the positive results of a single clinical trial in the case of beta-interferon, and one positive and one negative study for tissue plasminogen activator. Furthermore, the regulations provide for a lesser standard when the prospectively defined endpoint is survival. One part ('Subpart E') of the regulations specifically provides for an approval based on a single study if the drug has been shown to be safe and has a statistically significant impact on survival. Under that regulation, the definition of survival also extends to its surrogates, including tracheostomy.

By far the most comprehensive reforms in FDA regulations were driven by clinical trials in patients suffering from AIDS. In this context, the agency has written regulations ('Subpart H') that permit the use of surrogate endpoints (e.g. CD4 counts in patients with AIDS) as valid endpoints in clinical research. A statistically significant effect on a surrogate endpoint in the context of an acceptable risk profile is often sufficient for approval. Additional studies are required after approval in an attempt to move beyond the surrogate endpoints and to obtain data with well accepted clinical endpoints that may require years to acquire. Although the Subpart H regulations have been used to approve nonAIDS-related products (e.g. oncology products), they have not yet found utility in approving products for neurological disorders, because valid surrogate markers for MND and other seriously debilitating and neurological disorders have not yet been fully defined and validated. The limitations of the Subpart H regulations in neurological disease was specifically relieved in the FDA Reform Act of 1997. The new 'fast track' provision stipulates that in lieu of surrogate endpoints a clinical endpoint can be used to support a single-study approval in life threatening or seriously disabling diseases such as MND. Trialists, the pharmaceutical industry, and MND patients in the USA await the implementation of these new federally-mandated standards for promising new therapies of MND.

A 1996 guidance document was published by the FDA which provided other alternatives for single-study approvals for debilitating diseases such as MND. The guidance largely speaks to independent evidence within a single study that can be used to corroborate the results of the primary endpoint. This guideline has been used to approve interferon-β1 for multiple sclerosis, in which the effects of the drug on clinical endpoints were independently corroborated by quantitative MRI which correlated a decrease in the number of CNS lesions with the measured clinical benefit in the same clinical study.

On the surface, these new regulations and guidance appear to provide for a more cost effective path toward approval for serious orphan diseases. However, the interpretation of these regulations varies across divisions and among individuals within the FDA. It will be crucial for patients with ALS that among the divisions considering marketing applications for new drugs, interpretation of the Orphan Drug Act and the internal FDA guidance is applied uniformly. Further clarification of these important issues will be instrumental in fostering continued corporate interest in orphan diseases.

Expectations

New technology and a resurgent interest in MND has raised expectations that therapeutics which produce meaningful clinical effects will find their way into clinical practice. While anything less than a cure is met with disappointment, we need to consider how few neurological illnesses are cured. A 10–35% change in disease outcome is currently the state of the art for most neurological illnesses that are treated today (Table 8.3).

At face value, a 10–35% treatment effect may appear modest, but this magnitude of effect must be considered within the context of the particular disease state and the study population. In the rhIGF-1 study a mean reduction in disease progression of 25% occurred within a range of response from zero in some patients to greater than 90% in others. This consideration is particularly salient in chronic neurodegenerative diseases such as MND, in which symptom development may be latent and disease progression to increasingly morbid states is rapid and unrelenting. For example, several studies (Wohlfart, 1957; Sobue et al., 1983; Dantes and McComas, 1991; Felice, 1995) have suggested that, on average, half of lower motor neurons are lost before the appearance of the initial clinical symptoms, usually muscle weakness. These results are similar to those observed in Parkinson's disease where it has been reported that approximately 80% of striatal dopamine (Bernheimer et al., 1973) and 50% of the neurons in the substantia nigra (Fearnley and Lees, 1991) are lost before the appearance of extrapyramidal symptoms. Because neurons in the adult central nervous system have little, if any, capacity to regenerate, there is little hope that any therapeutic option will reverse the course of MND. However, a pharmaceutical agent that promotes neuron survival and retards the continous degenerative process (disease modifying) and/or enhances the patient's regenerative response to this disease would be predicted to demonstrate a therapeutic benefit by slowing the progression of muscle deterioration. Transplantation therapies, which are being explored for advanced Parkinson's patients, are less likely to offer meaningful outcomes in MND, in which all levels of the neuraxis (spinal cord, brainstem, and motor cortex) are involved (but see Chapter 9).

The latency to detectable muscle deterioration in patients with MND, despite the extensive degeneration of motor neurons, may be explained by the enormous capacity of peripheral motor nerves to collateralize and reinnervate denervated muscle fibers, which partially sustains muscle strength and func-

Table 8.3 Magnitude of treatment effects in neurological disorders

Disorder	Treatment	Treatment effect	Reference
Duchenne muscular dystrophy	Prednisone	approximately 10% improvement in muscle strength	Mendell et al., 1989; Griggs et al., 1991
Relapsing remitting MS	Interferon β-1b	34% decrease in relapse rate	IFNB Multiple Sclerosis Study Group, 1993
Parkinson's disease	Pramipexole	22–25% improvement in UPDRS II and III disability scores	Lieberman et al., 1997
ALS	Riluzole	28% increase in survival at 12 months	Bensimon et al., 1994

tion. The collateralization of motor neuron fibers is apparently so extensive in MND patients that the normal innervation ratio of motor neurons to muscle fibers is increased by 2–3-fold (Coers et al., 1973). The rapid deterioration of muscle function after the onset of symptoms is driven by the loss of these broadly collateralized neurons. In fact, the functioning motor unit population is halved in each 6-month period in the first year following diagnosis (Dantes and McComas, 1991); that is, the loss of motor units is logarithmic in this stage of disease. Because each collateralized motor neuron controls an extensive field of muscle fibers, even if a drug candidate were to rescue the majority of motor neurons, the loss of even a small fraction of neurons would have a significant negative impact on overall muscle function. Thus, the magnitude of effect of a therapeutic agent which reduces the rate of motor neuron death is likely to be minimized by the exponential loss of motor units which is so characteristic of MND.

Clinical studies have shown that both nodal and junctional sprouting occur in MND patients (Bjornskov et al., 1984). This increase in the number of sprouts is accompanied by an increase in nerve fiber density (Stahlberg et al., 1975) and is correlated with an increase in the size of the motor unit (Dantes and McComas, 1991). In this manner, MND patients compensate to some degree for the loss of their spinal motor neurons. Modification of motor end plates (Bjornskov et al., 1975) continues until the number of remaining motor neurons is no longer sufficient to reinnervate muscle and symptoms begin to appear (Wohlfart, 1957). When fewer than 5% of the motor neurons remain, sprouting and regeneration virtually cease (Hansen and Ballantyne, 1978). Although both forms of sprouting continue late into the disease process, there is a finite opportunity for a therapeutic agent to effect further sprouting in more advanced stage patients. Thus, the magnitude of effect of an agent that induces peripheral nerve sprouting would be muted in those patients whose surviving motor neurons are approaching the limits of their regenerative capacity. One simple way of viewing progression of MND is that it is a balance of motor neuron degeneration and peripheral motor nerve regeneration.

The magnitude of any treatment effect must be interpreted in the context of what is possible to achieve in the study population. Once motor neurons have degenerated they cannot regenerate. Therefore, any expectation that drug intervention will reverse the progression of MND will probably go unfulfilled. Moreover, the magnitude of a drug effect on the nervous system is muted clinically by the exponential loss of muscle fibers. Only if *all* motor neuron degeneration were stopped abruptly, as might occur in poliomyelitis or the subacute motor neuron disease of lymphoma, could compensatory regeneration *regain* some function. This is the holy grail to be hoped for. The loss of most motor neurons and the extensive compensatory regenerative response in ALS before appearance of the first symptoms renders it difficult to conceive of a large effect on muscle function in a population at varying clinical stages of disease. Therefore, any measurable effect must be interpreted as clinically meaningful in the context of *this* disease. Of course, one might speculate that a greater response may be achieved in MND patients if therapy were initiated before the appearance of the first symptom, a possibility currently only in rare pedigrees of familial ALS.

Summary

The resurgent interest in MND has been driven by scientific developments in the 1990s. Important insights into the cellular and molecular mechanisms of motor neuron death gleaned from basic research has allowed for a more mechanistic approach to clinical research.

The successes and failures of clinical trials in this field have highlighted important variables, which, if not properly controlled for, will yield largely uninterpretable and equivocal clinical results.

Incentives to induce continued investment in clinical research in the form of recently modified orphan drug laws and a favorable international regulatory environment appear to be properly aligned with the interests of patients, physicians, and corporate sponsors of research.

As in all areas of discovery research, success will breed followers. The notable successes in both basic and clinical research will be a powerful motivational force to advance our understanding and treatment of MND.

References

Adem A, Ekblom J, Gillberg PG et al. (1994) Insulin-like growth factor-1 receptors in human spinal cord: changes in amyotrophic lateral sclerosis. J Neural Transm 97: 73–84.

ALS CNTF Treatment Study (ACTS) Phase I-II Study Group (1995) A phase I study of recombinant human ciliary neurotrophic factor (RHCNTF) in patients with amyotrophic lateral sclerosis. Clin Neuropharmacol 18: 515–532.

ALS CNTF Treatment Study (ACTS) Phase I-II Study Group (1996a) The amyotrophic lateral sclerosis functional rating scale – assessment of activities of daily living in patients with amyotrophic lateral sclerosis. Arch Neurol 53: 141–147.

ALS CNTF Treatment Study (ACTS) Phase II-III Study Group (1996b) A double-blind placebo-controlled clinical trial of subcutaneous recombinant human ciliary neurotrophic factor (RHCNTF) in amyotrophic lateral sclerosis. Neurology 46: 1244–1249.

Andres PL, Hedlund W, Finison L et al. (1986) Quantitative motor assessment in amyotrophic lateral sclerosis. Neurology 36: 937–941.

Appel SH (1993) Excitotoxic neuronal cell death in amyotrophic lateral sclerosis. Trends Neurosci 16: 3–5.

Appel V, Stewart SS, Smith G et al. (1987) A rating scale for amyotrophic lateral sclerosis: description and preliminary experience. Ann Neurol 22: 328–333.

BDNF Study Group (Phase III) (1999) A controlled trial of recombinant methionyl human BDNF in ALS. Neurology 52: 1427–1433.

Bensimon G, Lacomblez L, Meininger V, and the ALS/Riluzole Study Group (1994) A controlled trial of riluzole in amyotrophic lateral sclerosis. N Engl J Med 330: 585–591.

Bernheimer H, Birkmayer W, Hornykiewicz O et al. (1973) Brain dopamine and the syndromes of Parkinson and Huntington: clinical, morphological and neurochemical correlations. J Neurol Sci 20: 415–455.

Bjornskov EK, Dekker NP, Norris FH et al. (1975) End-plate morphology in amyotrophic lateral sclerosis. Arch Neurol 32: 711–712.

Bjornskov EK, Norris FH, Mower-Kuby J (1984) Quantitative axon terminal and end-plate morphology in amyotrophic lateral sclerosis. Arch Neurol 41: 527–530.

Borasio GD, Robberecht W, Leigh PN et al. (1998) A placebo-controlled trial of insulin-like growth factor-I in amyotrophic lateral sclerosis. Neurology 51: 583–586.

Bohn MC (1999) A commentary on glial cell line-derived neurotrophic factor (GDNF). From a glial secreted molecule to gene therapy. Biochem Pharmacol 57: 135–142.

Bossuyt PM, Louwerse ES, Weverling GJ, de Jong JMBV (1995) Baseline assessments in amyotrophic lateral sclerosis trials. J Neurol Sci 129 (Suppl): 28.

Brooks BR (1994) The Norris ALS score: insight into the natural history of amyotrophic lateral sclerosis provided by Forbes Norris. In: Rose FC (ed). ALS – From Charcot to the Present and into the Future – The Forbes H. Norris (1928–1993) Memorial Volume. Smith-Gordon: London, pp. 21–29.

Brooks BR (1996a) A double-blind placebo-controlled clinical trial of subcutaneous recombinant human ciliary neurotrophic factor (rHCNTF) in amyotrophic lateral sclerosis. Neurology 46: 1244–1249.

Brooks BR (1996b) Natural history of ALS: symptoms, strength, pulmonary function, and disability. Neurology 47(Suppl 2): S71–S82.

Brooks BR, Lewis D, Rawling J et al. (1994) The natural history of amyotrophic lateral sclerosis. In: William AC (ed.) Motor Neuron Disease. Chapman & Hall: London, pp. 131–169.

Brooks BR, Sufit RL, DePaul R et al. (1991) Design of clinical therapeutic trials in amyotrophic lateral sclerosis. Adv Neurol 56: 521–546.

Caroni P, Grandes P (1990) Nerve sprouting in innervated adult skeletal muscle induced by exposure to elevated levels of insulin-like growth factors. J Cell Biol 110: 1307–1317.

Cedarbaum JM, Mitsumoto H et al. (2000) An open-label safety and tolerability study of high-dose subcutaneous recombinant methionyl-human brain derived neurotrophic factor in 30 patients with ALS. Neurology 54(Suppl 3): 342–343.

Coërs C, Telerman-Toppet N, Gerard JM (1973) Terminal innervation ratio in neuromuscular diseases: II. Disorders of lower motor neuron, peripheral nerve, and muscle. Arch Neurol 49: 215–222.

Contreras PC, Steffler C, Yu E, Callison K, Strong D, Vaught JL (1995) Systemic administration of rhIGF-I enhanced regeneration after sciatic nerve crush in mice. J Pharmacol Exp Ther 274: 1443–1449.

Corse AM, Bilak MM, Bilak SR, Lehar M, Rothstein JD, Kuncl RW (1999) Preclinical testing of neuroprotective neurotrophic factors in a model of chronic motor neuron degeneration. Neurobiol Dis 6: 335–346.

Cudkowicz ME, Warren L, Francis JW et al. (1997) Intrathecal administration of recombinant human superoxide dismutase 1 in amyotrophic lateral sclerosis: a preliminary safety and pharmacokinetic study. Neurology 49: 213–222.

Deng H-X, Hentati A, Tainer JA et al. (1993) Amyotrophic lateral sclerosis and structural defects in Cu, Zn superoxide dismutase. Science 261: 1047–1051.

Doré S, Kar S, Quirion R (1997) Rediscovering an old friend, IGF-I: potential use in the treatment of neurodegenerative diseases. Trends Neurosci 20: 326–331.

Drachman DB, Chaudhry V, Cornblath D et al. (1994) Trial of immunosuppression in amyotrophic lateral sclerosis using total lymphoid irradiation. Ann Neurol 35: 142–150.

European parliament committee unanimously accepts common position on orphan drugs. Int Pharmaceut Regul Monitor 27 (12);3 (Suppl F – Council of Ministers' Common Position on Orphan Drugs).

Fearnley JM, Lees AJ (1991) Aging and Parkinson's disease: substantia nigra regional selectivity. Brain 114: 2283–2301.

Felice KJ (1995) Thenar motor unit number estimates using the multiple point stimulation technique: reproducibility studies in ALS patients and normal subjects. Muscle Nerve 18: 1412–1416.

Felice KJ (1997) A longitudinal study comparing thenar motor unit number estimates to other quantitative tests in patients with ALS. Muscle Nerve 20: 179–185.

Gooch CL, Harati Y (2000) Motor unit number estimation, ALS and clinical trials. ALS 1: 71–82.

Griggs RC, Moxley RT, Mendell JR et al. Clinical Investigation of Duchenne Dystrophy Group (1991) Prednisone in Duchenne dystrophy: a randomized, controlled trial defining the time course and dose response. Arch Neurol 48: 383–388.

Gurney ME, Pu H, Chiu AY et al. (1994) Motor neuron degeneration in mice that express a human Cu,Zn superoxide dismutase mutation. Science 264: 1772–1775.

Gurney ME, Cutting FB, Zhai P et al. (1996) Benefit of vitamin E, riluzole, and gabapentin in a transgenic model of familial amyotrophic lateral sclerosis. Ann Neurol 39: 147–157.

Hansson H.A., Dahlin LB, Danielsen N et al. (1985) Evidence indicating trophic importance of IGF-I in regenerating peripheral nerves. Acta Physiol Scand 126: 609–614.

Haverkamp LJ, Appel V, Appel SH (1995) Natural history of amyotrophic lateral sclerosis in a database population: validation of a scoring system and a model for survival prediction. Brain 118: 707–719.

IFNB Multiple Sclerosis Study Group (1993) Interferon beta-1b is effective in relapsing-remitting multiple sclerosis. I. Clinical results of a multi-center, randomized, double-blind, placebo-controlled trial. Neurology 43: 655–661.

Kanje M, Skottner A, Lundborg G et al. (1991) Does insulin-like growth factor I (IGF-1) trigger the cell body reaction in the rat sciatic nerve? Brain Research 563: 285–287.

Kiernan JA, Hudson JA (1993) Anti-neurone antibodies are not characteristic of amyotrophic lateral sclerosis. Neuro Report 4: 427–430.

Lacomblez L, Bensimon G, Leigh PG et al. (1996): Dose-ranging study of riluzole in amyotrophic lateral sclerosis. Lancet 347: 1425–1431.

Lai EC, Felice KJ, Festoff BW et al. (1997) Effect of recombinant insulin-like growth factor-1 on progression of ALS; a placebo controlled study. Neurology 49: 1621–1630.

Lewis ME, Neff NT, Contreras PC et al. (1993) Insulin-like growth factor-I: potential for treatment of motor neuronal disorders. Exp Neurol 124: 73–88.

Lieberman A, Ranhosky A, Korts D (1997) Clinical evaluation of pramipexole in advanced Parkinson's disease: results of a double-blind, placebo-controlled, parallel-group study. Neurology 49: 162–168.

Louwerse ES, Bossuyt PMM, Weverling GJ, de Jong JMBV (1996) Baseline assessments in therapeutic trials in amyotrophic lateral sclerosis. In Louwerse ES Amyotrophic Lateral Sclerosis: Clinical and Methodological Studies (PhD dissertation). Delft: Van Marken Publishers, pp. 99–109. Abstract (1995) published in J Neurol Sci 129 (Suppl): 28.

Louwerse ES, Visser CE, Bossuyt PMM, Weverling GJ, The Netherlands ALS Consortium (1997): Amyotrophic lateral sclerosis: mortality risk during the course of the disease and prognostic factors. J Neurol Sci 152 (Suppl 1): S10–S17.

Mazzini L, Mora G, Balzarini C et al. (1998) The natural history and the effects of gabapentin in amyotrophic lateral sclerosis. J Neurol Sci 160(Suppl 1): S57–S63.

McNamara JO, Fridovich I (1993) Did radicals strike Lou Gehrig? Nature 362: 20–21.

Mendell JR, Moxley RT, Griggs RC et al. (1989) Randomized, double-blind six-month trial of prednisone in Duchenne's muscular dystrophy. N Engl J Med 320: 1592–1597.

Miller RG, Moore D, Young LA et al. (1996a) Placebo-controlled trial of gabapentin in patients with amyotrophic lateral sclerosis. Neurology 47: 1383–1388.

Miller RG, Shepherd R, Dao H et al. (1996b) Controlled trial of nimodipine in amyotrophic lateral sclerosis. Neuromusc Disord 4: 101–104.

Miller RG, Smith SA, Murphy JR et al. (1996c) A clinical trial of verapamil in amyotrophic lateral sclerosis. Muscle Nerve 19: 511–515.

Miller RG, Petajan JH, Bryan WW et al. (1996d) A placebo-controlled trial of recombinant human ciliary neurotrophic (rhCNTF) factor in amyotrophic lateral sclerosis. Ann Neurol 39: 256–260.

Mucke HAM, Castañer J (1998) SR-57746A: 5-HT$_{1A}$ receptor agonist nerve growth factor potentiator. Drugs Future 23: 616–619.

Munsat TL, Andres PL, Skerry LM (1989) The use of quantitative techniques to define amyotrophic lateral sclerosis. In: Munsat TL (ed.) Quantification of Neurologic Deficit. Butterworths: Boston, pp. 129–142.

Norris FH, Calanchini PR, Fallat R, Panchri S, Jewett BJ (1974) The administration of guanidine in amyotrophic lateral sclerosis. Neurology 24: 721–728.

Paty DW, Li DKB, UBC MS/MRI Study Group et al. (1993) Interferon beta-1b is effective in relapsing-remitting multiple sclerosis, II: MRI analysis results of a multicenter, randomized, double-blind, placebo-controlled trial. Neurol 43: 662–667.

Preux P-M, Couratier Ph, Boutros-Toni F et al. (1996) Survival prediction in sporadic amyotrophic lateral sclerosis: age and clinical form at onset are independent risk factors. Neuroepidemiology 15: 153–160.

Ringel SP, Murphy JR, Alderson MK et al. (1993) The natural history of amyotrophic lateral sclerosis. Neurology 43: 1316–1322.

Rosen DR, Siddique T, Patteson D et al. (1993) Mutations in Cu/Zn superoxide dismutase gene are associated with familial amyotrophic lateral sclerosis. Nature 362: 59–62.

Rothstein JD, Jin L, Dykes-Hoberg M, Kuncl RW (1993) Chronic inhibition of glutamate uptake produces a model of slow neurotoxicity. Proc Natl Acad Sci USA 90: 6591–6595.

Rothstein JD, Dykes-Hoberg M, Pardo CA et al. (1996) Antisense knockout of glutamate transporters reveals a predominant role for astroglial glutamate transport in excitotoxicity and clearance of extracellular glutamate. Neuron 16: 675–686.

Rothstein JD, Kuncl R, Chaudhry V et al. (1991) Excitatory amino acids in amyotrophic lateral sclerosis: An update. Ann Neurol 30: 224–245.

Rothstein JD, Martin L, Kuncl RW (1992) Decreased glutamate transport by the brain and spinal cord in amyotrophic lateral sclerosis. N Engl J Med 326: 1464–1468.

Rothstein JD, Van Kammen M, Levey AL et al. (1995) Selective loss of glial glutamate transporter GLT-1 in amyotrophic lateral sclerosis. Ann Neurol 38: 73–84.

Scrip Daily Online (1999) Gabapentin. Nov. 8.

Smith RA, Melmed S, Sherman B et al. (1993) Recombinant growth hormone treatment of amyotrophic lateral sclerosis. Muscle Nerve 16: 624–633.

Sobue G, Sahashi K, Takahashi A, Matsuoka Y, Muroga T, Sobue I (1983) Degenerating compartment and functioning compartment of motor neurons in ALS: possible process of motor neuron loss. Neurology 33: 654–657.

Stahlberg ES, Schwartz MS, Trontelj JV (1975) Single fibre electromyography in various processes affecting the anterior horn cell. J Neurol Sci 24: 403–415.

Winkler J, Thal LJ (1994) Clinical potential of growth factors in neurological disorders. CNS Drugs 6: 465–478.

Wohlfart G (1957) Collateral regeneration from residual motor nerve fibers in amyotrophic lateral sclerosis. Neurology 7: 124–134.

Future therapy of ALS and SMA

Andrew Eisen and William Jia

Introduction

Spinal muscular atrophy (SMA) is primarily a disorder of infancy and childhood, although adult onset cases do occur (see Chapter 5). On the other hand, amyotrophic lateral sclerosis (ALS) is a heterogeneous, multifactorial disease occurring on the background of an aging nervous system. Thus, the therapeutic challenges for the two disorders differ. The early onset of the spinal muscular atrophies raises at least two possible future therapeutic avenues: one is to replace defective genes, and the other is to modulate the abnormal gene product(s) that are presumed responsible for abnormal neuronal functioning. By contrast, ALS being a disease of the aging nervous system, requires early diagnosis for implementation of protective measures to prevent or modify normal neuronal aging and associated neuronal dysfunction or death. Presently, there is no ideal biological marker for sporadic ALS so that early identification of those who might be at risk is difficult. When a marker that is highly disease specific becomes available, early therapeutic intervention will become possible. Problems related to early detection apply equally to other neurodegenerative disorders and most cancers. Advances in mapping of genomes have made it feasible to search among the anonymous polygenes of complex systems for loci of intermediate effect size (quantitative trait loci). This will open the possibility of exploring the genetic architecture and the anatomical, physiological, biochemical, and molecular mechanisms underlying specific disease phenotypes (McClearn, 1997).

As implied in its title, this chapter is largely speculative, and to what extent any of the therapies explored will become reality only time will tell. Nevertheless, for ALS and SMA, this is an exciting time. Within the last decade, there has been an explosion in the understanding of the fundamental principles underlying these diseases, and meaningful therapy that significantly adds to the quality of life cannot be far away.

Spinal muscular atrophy

SMA spares the upper motor neuron, which makes it distinct from ALS. Overall, nearly 99% of patients have an absent or abnormality of the survival motor neuron gene (*SMN*). More than 95% of cases of SMA have an undetectable survival motor neuron gene which is located on human chromosome 5 (5q12-q13) (Brzustowicz et al., 1990; Melki et al., 1990; Morrison, 1996). In a small percentage, this gene is present but partially deleted, and in a few other cases there are disabling point mutations within the coding region of the gene (reviewed in Crawford, 1996). The full-length form of the neuronal apoptosis inhibitor protein gene is deleted in about 45% of SMA type 1 and around 18% of SMA type 2 (reviewed in Crawford, 1996). Programmed death of motor neurons (apoptosis) is a normal phenomenon during embryogenesis, and one model of SMA invokes an inappropriate persistence of motor neuron apoptosis. The neuronal apoptosis inhibitory protein gene is responsible for the timely cessation of apoptosis in motor neurons (Roy et al., 1995).

The identification of *SMN* as the pathogenetic gene in spinal muscular atrophy not only facilitates the accurate genetic diagnosis of SMA but sets the stage for directed gene therapy. Gene therapy is best defined as the provision of a gene, the product of which can alleviate the consequences of a pathological condition (Kay and Woo, 1994). Barriers to success are formidable. A suitable vector that can stably introduce activated and intact copies of the abnormal genes identified in SMA into the motor neurons will need to be developed. Replacement therapy would have to occur in a timely fashion in order to stop motor neuron loss. Therefore, upregulation of *SMN* by either genetic or pharmacologic means is the thrust of current experimental therapeutic approaches.

Viral vectors for gene therapy, as detailed below, are still problematic. In terms of treating SMA the gene constructs would have to reach motor neurons diffusely in a multisegmental fashion. It has been shown experimentally that it is possible to deliver plasmid gene constructs directly into spinal motor neurons utilizing retrograde axoplasmic transport after injection into the sciatic nerve or gastrocnemius muscle (Sahenk et al., 1993). This is not practical in a diffuse, multisegmental anterior horn cell disease, and transplantation of progenitor (stem-like) cells would be preferable. This approach is described below for ALS. It would also be reasonable to use the same viral vector to introduce one or more growth factors to maintain 'healthy' or functioning spinal motor neurons and thereby help promote sprouting of their axons. Adenovirus-mediated gene transfer of neurotrophin-3 produces substantial therapeutic effects in the mouse progressive motor neuronopathy, with a 50% increase in life span, reduced loss of motor axons, and improved neuromuscular function (Haase et al., 1997). The benefits can be further enhanced by co-injecting an adenoviral vector coding for ciliary neurotrophic factor.

It is thought that the neuronal apoptosis inhibitory protein gene retards naturally occurring embryogenesis and early life apoptosis, and mutations in this gene might contribute to excessive apoptosis and motor neuron loss. Anti-apoptotic strategies are rational to counteract any deleterious effects of altered neuronal apoptosis inhibitory protein function in SMA. Anti-apoptotic therapy is discussed below.

ALS future therapeutic strategies

Several approaches that have potential application for treating ALS will be outlined. They are not mutually exclusive and indeed share important fundamentals so that two or more might be simultaneously implemented.

Protecting the aging genome

With aging, genetic information becomes subject to random errors, and damage to informational molecules occurs (Rattan, 1995). Normally functioning cells are reduced in number below a critical level for physiological functioning in many systems, including the motor system, which puts added burden on surviving cells. This is likely of relevance in the pre-clinical stage of ALS that later cascades into a series of events leading to neuronal death and clinically overt ALS. Some of the age-related gene degradation follows a combination of chronic oxidative stress from the accumulation of reactive oxygen species (Hockenbery et al., 1993; Veis et al., 1993; Simonian and Coyle, 1996), mitochondrial failure (Beal, 1995; Johns, 1996), glutamatergic excitotoxicity (Rothstein, 1995), damage to vital organelles, and aberrant protein aggregation. Other mechanisms are yet to be clarified (Eisen et al., 1995; Eisen and Krieger, 1998). Current therapeutic efforts in ALS, which at best have been very modest, have been largely directed to counteracting these pre-terminal events.

The human genome is now estimated to have between 30,000 and 40,000 genes (Venter et al., 2001). Specific genes are directly responsible for maintenance of cell function and some are protective against 'neuronal aging'. Now that the sequence of the human genome is virtually complete it should become possible to identify 'candidate pathways' in aging and longevity by comparing groups of elderly individuals with select phenotypes for sequence variation. (Vijg and van Orsouw, 2002). Bio-gerontology is the study of the aging of biological systems. The rate of random chemical damage to the genome is considered the major factor determining lifespan of species. Oxidative stress and reactive oxygen species are recognized as a primary source of damage in aging and chronic disease, inducing silent cumulative damage to the genome as a consequence of imperfect repair. Future studies will have to focus on the effects of inhibitors of genomic damage and lifespan extension (Baynes, 2000).

Since only a small subset of ALS can be attributed to one particular molecular defect (such as mutation of *SOD1* or the gene encoding neurofilament H), the etiology of ALS is likely to be multifactorial. A search is needed for specific susceptibility genes rendering particular individuals at greater risk for developing ALS. This would make it possible to appropriately initiate some therapies such as glutamate antagonists and antioxidants in the pre-clinical stages of ALS, somewhat akin to the administration of aspirin to prevent heart disease and stroke in susceptible individuals. Eventually, it will become possible to modify susceptibility genes that would allow more direct protection against neuronal aging and damage. Identification of susceptibility genes is already proving invaluable in other diseases such as breast and colonic cancer. Definitive susceptibility or protective genes have not been identified for ALS and one can only guess at a number of possible candidates that may play a role in ALS. Given the considerable phenotypic heterogeneity of the disease such as its age of onset, rate of progression, and site of onset and spread of deficit, there must be many relevant susceptibility (or protective) genes in ALS. Some possible candidates for the sporadic disease include the Cu/Zn *SOD-1* gene, the P2 blood group gene, the neurofilament heavy gene (Figlewicz et al., 1994; Al-Chalabi et al., 1995; Julien, 1995), *SMN1* and *SMN2* (Moulard et al., 1998; Veldink et al., 2001; Corcia et al., 2002), possibly the parvalbumin gene (Ince et al., 1993), and maybe telomeric DNA (Harley, 1997; Dahse et al., 1997; Greider, 1998).

Telomerase replacement

Vertebrates have special structures at the ends of their chromosomes, known as telomeres. They are composed of 5- to 15-kb pairs of a guanine-rich hexameric repeats (Landman et al., 1997). With aging, there is a progressive degradation of telomeres in normal somatic cells and neuronal precursors (Kruk et al., 1996; Steinert et al., 2002). The cell can afford to lose only a finite number of telomeres before significant parent DNA sequences are lost (Vaziri and Benchimol, 1998). When this occurs, there is chromosomal instability and the cell dies. However, germ-cell telomeres are maintained despite multiple rounds of replication, which suggests that they produce products that maintain telomere length. Telomerase, an enzymatic ribonucleoprotein, appears to be essential in maintenance of telomere length and it is necessary for cellular immortalization (Zakian, 1995; Yanagi et al., 1997). Erosion of telomeric DNA appears to be due to the lack of expression of components of the telomere maintenance system and this limits the replicative capacity of cells, shortening the lifespan of key systems in the body (Morin, 1997). Loss of telomeric DNA is then key to neuronal aging (Dahse et al., 1997; Harley, 1997; Greider, 1998). The lifespan of cultured cells is dependent on the age of the individual donor, and it has been shown that telomerase expression stabilizes telomere length and allows for continual replication so that viable chromosomes can be transmitted to the next generation (Harley and Sherwood, 1997). In the future, it may be possible to genetically engineer vectors that can 'replenish' the telomere maintenance system. Telomerse activity has been shown to be restored in human cells by ectopic expression of human telomerase reverse transcriptase (hTERT, hEST2) (Counter et al., 1998). The telomere maintenance system must be closely linked to nuclear and mitochondrial DNA repair mechanisms which too are crucial determinants of a cell's lifespan (Cortopassi and Wang, 1996). Comparative studies of DNA repair in different species shows a good correlation between DNA repair activity and lifespan, with nonhuman primates having an approximately six-fold relative DNA repair activity compared to that of small mammals (Cortopassi and Wang, 1996).

Substantial research efforts have focused on the transcriptional regulation of the catalytic protein component of telomerase, hTERT. However, increasing evidence indicates that regulation of hTERT is complex, and much remains to be learned about the regulation of telomerase. Generation of full-length hTERT protein is likely to be the limiting step in the formation of active telomerase. Regulation of hTERT transcription, transport to the nucleus, assembly of the telomerase holoenzyme, recruitment of telomerase to the telomere, and the role of post-translational modifications of hTERT protein are areas of intense investigation. It is hoped that shedding light on these diverse areas of telomerase regulation will eventually allow manipulation of telomerase activity for therapeutic purposes (Aisner et al., 2002).

Gene therapy using viral vectors in ALS

The essence of gene therapy for ALS would require transfer of gene products into the CNS, to positively influence neuronal populations that are selectively vulnerable. The ideal vector must embody levels of gene expression or drug which can be regulated and controlled and must specifically target those neurons primarily involved in ALS. This includes both the corticomotoneurons in the motor cortex and the spinal anterior horn cells. But, other cells, such as local-circuit inhibitory interneurons and glial cells, may be important. Ideally, the vectors should have long-term gene expression following single injections.

In the last decade adenovirus vectors have emerged as promising technology in gene therapy. They have been used for genetic modification of a variety of somatic cells in vitro and in vivo. They have been widely used as gene delivery vectors in experiments both with curative and preventive purposes. Adenovirus vectors have been used in the experimental and in some extent in the clinical gene therapy of several cancers. The combination of recombinant adenovirus technology with chemotherapy (pro drug system) seems to be promising, too. Adenovirus vectors offer several advantages over other vectors. Replication defective vectors can be produced in very high titers (10 pfu/ml) thus allowing a substantially greater efficiency of direct gene transfer; they have the capacity to infect both replicating and non-replicating (quiescent) cells from a variety of tissues and species. Several important limitations of adenovirus-mediated gene transfer are also known, such as the relatively short-term (transient) expression of foreign genes, induction of the host humeral and cellular immune response to viral proteins and viral infected cells, which may substantially inhibit the effect of repeated treatment with adenovirus vectors, the limited cloning capacity, and the lack of target cell specificity. However, the well-understood structure, molecular biology and host cell interactions of adenoviruses offer some potential solutions to these limitations (Nasz and Adam, 2001).

Neural progenitor cells may provide for cell replacement or gene delivery vehicles in the therapy of neurodegenerative disease. The expression of therapeutic proteins by neural progenitors would be enhanced by viral-mediated gene transfer, but the effects of several common recombinant viruses on primary progenitor cell populations have not been extensively tested. Hughes et al. (2002) have shown that feline immunodeficiency virus, adeno-associated virus or adenovirus can all transduce progenitor cell populations in vitro, with maintenance of their ability to differentiate into multiple cell types or to respond to injury within the central nervous system. Such results hold promise for the use of genetically manipulated stem cells for CNS therapies. One of the major challenges for gene therapy is systemic delivery of a nucleic acid directly into an affected tissue. This requires developing a vehicle which is able to protect the nucleic acid from degradation, while delivering the gene of interest to the specific tissue and specific sub-cellular compartment. This might be better accomplished through non-viral delivery systems. Two types of gene delivery systems, LPD1 (cationic liposome-entrapped, polycation-condensed DNA, type 1), and retention-time mediated naked DNA delivery, have recently been described (Liu and Huang, 2002).

Currently available delivery systems commonly used for transferring genes into cells include cationic liposomes and several viral vectors. Cationic liposomes have been widely used for transferring genes into cultured cells in vitro (Felgner et al., 1994; Sorscher et al., 1994; Yagi et al., 1994; Puyal et al., 1995; Rosenblum and Chen, 1995). Despite some progress, the in vitro transfection efficiency of cationic liposomes is still unsatisfactory compared with viral vector systems, which remain the most efficient means for gene delivery in vivo (Kasahara et al., 1994).

Three viral systems are commonly used for gene delivery (Robbins et al., 1998):

- Retrovirus (Gunzburg et al., 1996)
- Adenovirus (including adeno-associate virus) (Peltekian et al., 1997; Davidson and Bohn, 1997; Snoeck et al., 1997)
- Herpes virus (Glorioso et al., 1994).

Retroviral and adenoviral vectors have been used to deliver genes in a variety of experimental animal models for the therapy of both nervous and non-nervous system disorders. Recent clinical trials have commenced with herpes virus as a vector for gene delivery in the treatment of brain tumors. Herpes virus has neurotrophic properties that add particular advantage to its use in treating central nervous system disorders.

The expression of genes that are delivered via a retroviral vector requires at least one mitotic cycle of the target cell. Thus, in adult brain therapy, using retroviral vectors is restricted to nonneuronal cells. Unlike adenovirus and herpes virus, which are DNA viruses, retrovirus vectors insert themselves into the genome of host cells. As a result, the gene transfer is permanent and the gene is likely to be carried by many generations of the transduced cells. With retroviral vectors, there is the difficulty of obtaining a high-titer virus stock because of the low efficiency of propagation within cultured cells. There is a limited spread within the host and this precludes infection of a large number of cells in vivo. Retroviral vectors are thus the most useful for generating genetically engineered neuronal progenitor cells that, as described later, can be injected into the adult central nervous system and potentially differentiate into functional neurons once transplanted into CNS.

The infective titer of adenoviral vectors is several orders of magnitude higher than that of retroviral vectors. In the brain, adenovirus can readily infect a variety of cells with very high efficiency. Adenovirus vectors have been used to deliver a variety of genes into the CNS for gene therapy in animal models. Examples are β-glucuronidase (Ohashi et al., 1997), interleukins (Brauner et al., 1997; Bui et al., 1997; Felzmann et al., 1997; Emtage et al., 1998), neurotransmitter receptors (Ghavami et al., 1997; O'Connor et al., 1997; Umegaki et al., 1997), tyrosine hydroxylase (Mallet, 1996; Horellou and Mallet, 1997b), a bcl-2 viral vector protecting neurons from excitotoxicity (Jia, 1995), and a variety of neurotrophic factors (Baumgartner and Shine, 1997; Bilang et al., 1997; Gimenez et al., 1997; Gravel et al., 1997; Horellou and Mallet, 1997a).

However, there are disadvantages to using adenoviral vectors. They induce cytotoxicity in neurons which is due to the viral envelope proteins that can cause a severe inflammatory response. There are also other viral proteins that may be toxic to infected neurons. It is commonly believed that adenoviral vectors can accommodate foreign genes only if they are no larger than 7 kb. Although this size may be adequate for current gene therapies, it may be a problem in the future, considering that many human genes are much larger.

Herpes simplex virus type-1 (HSV-1) vector possesses some unique features that make it attractive (Glorioso et al., 1994; Roizman, 1996). The large genome of HSV-1 contains many nonessential genes that can be replaced. This allows insertion of multiple therapeutic genes that can be delivered using a single viral vector. HSV-1 virus is highly infectious to many cell types regardless of the phase of the cell cycle. More importantly, as a neurotrophic virus, HSV-1 can establish a latency in neurons and maintain the integrity of its genome for the lifetime of the host. This feature provides the possibility of long-term expression of a therapeutic gene in neuronal cells infected with HSV-1. Despite current failures in such long-term expression of foreign genes in animal models, it can be anticipated that, with growing knowledge of herpes virology and mechanism of latency, permanent expression of genes within neurons using HSV-1 as a vector can be achieved. However, HSV vectors do have drawbacks. HSV-1 has a more complex genome compared to the other two viral vectors. Like adenovirus, the cytotoxicity is still an important issue that requires detailed investigation when such viral vectors are used in vivo.

A common obstacle for viral mediated gene therapy in the treatment of CNS disorders is the poor dissemination of viral particles in the parenchyma (Fisher and Ray, 1994). Whereas biological delivery of a gene into a target cell can be very efficient, once a virus contacts the cell, physical spreading of viral particles themselves is rather poor in brain tissue. This limited physical diffusibility renders an anatomical specificity which is advantageous when localized gene delivery is required. On the other hand, it challenges the application of this technology in diseases involving neural damage that is widespread, extending along the entire neuraxis, as is the case in ALS and the spinal muscular atrophies. This problem can be circumvented to some extent when the vector is used to carry genes that encode for diffusible proteins such as growth factors. In these circumstances, the vector can be designed to target ventricular ependymal cells by intraventricular injection. Infection of ependymal cells with the viral vectors may result in the synthesis of sufficiently large quantities of the therapeutic protein, which when secreted into the cerebrospinal fluid will reach neurons on a global scale. However, different strategies will be needed to infuse sick neurons with other drugs, replace genes such as those needed for telomere maintenance, modify other genes such as susceptibility genes, or add protective genes.

Delivery of growth factors using viral vectors

Despite the relative failure demonstrated by neuronal growth factors in the treatment of ALS so far, the approach is rational and continues to hold appeal

(Seeburger and Springer, 1993; Apfel, 2002). Failure up to now may largely reflect an inadequate delivery system. A good example is the subcutaneous delivery of recombinant human ciliary neurotrophic factor (rhCNTF) in humans (Miller et al., 1996). This was frustrated by:

1) Peripheral side effects,
2) The molecule's short half-life (probably minutes), which is too short a time to induce a significant effect,
3) Its inability to cross the blood–brain barrier, resulting in very low-level concentrations of drug in the cerebrospinal fluid (CSF) and presumably target neurons.
4) Large doses of trophic factors given by injection, especially the cytokines, are toxic.

These problems can be overcome using appropriately encoded viral vectors. For example, adenovirus encoding brain-derived neurotrophic factor (BDNF) and the glial-cell line-derived neurotrophic factor (GDNF) have been administered by intramuscular injection. The trophic factors are taken up by retrograde axonal transport and incorporated into anterior horn cells (Gimenez et al., 1997). This strategy has been used experimentally in newborn rats to prevent the usual massive death of motoneurons that normally follows axotomy in the neonatal period. In the animals pre-treated with adenovirus encoding trophic factors, motoneuron survival is significantly increased. In the setting of ALS, this approach clearly has limitations. It would require repeated multisegmental injections, which would be unacceptable.

A related, and better approach, is to use polymer encapsulation of cells which have been genetically engineered to release one or more neurotrophic factors or other drugs into the central nervous system (Aebischer et al., 1996). The polymer-encapsulated cells can be implanted subcutaneously, intrathecally, and, as alluded to above, even intraventricularly. This method permits a continuous and slow release of neurotrophic factors in known concentrations. There is no fear of cell rejection because the semipermeable membrane isolates the cells. Similarly, there is no risk of tumor formation, and the polymer device can be removed in the event of a problem. Unfortunately these approaches have not proven useful in clinical trials.

It is also possible to inject cells genetically engineered to produce growth factors directly into the brain. For example, in a rat model of Parkinson's disease induced by intrastriatal injection of 6-hydroxydopamine, 60–70% of nigrostriatal neurons degenerate. Intrastriatal grafts of fibroblasts genetically engineered to produce BDNF partially prevented the loss of nerve terminals and completely prevented the loss of cell bodies of the nigrostriatal dopaminergic pathway. In contrast, the implantation of control fibroblasts that did not produce BDNF failed to protect nerve terminals and cell bodies. Similarly, GDNF expressing recombinant adenovirus injected into hindlimb muscles of neonatal *SOD-1* mice improved survival and function compared to control animals (Ascadi et al., 2001).

Anti-apoptotic strategies

Apoptosis (programmed cell death) is distinct from necrosis. It is controlled by a genetically active process that removes unwanted or damaged cells.

Apoptosis is an important regressive event during the normal development of the nervous system. For example, in the chick, mouse, rat, and human, approximately 50% of post-mitotic neurons die naturally during embryonic or fetal development by apoptosis (Kaal et al., 1997). It is possible to influence apoptosis so that there is over- or underexpression of the various genes that control the process. Some genes, such as the proto-oncogene *Bcl-2*, function as survival genes (under-expression of apoptosis) (Murphy et al., 1996) and others such as *ced3* or interleukin converting enzyme function as killer genes (overexpression of apoptosis).

Apoptosis is a multistep process controlled by the activation of unique gene expression. Apoptosis-associated genes can be categorized into four groups. There are those that provide signals to initiate apoptosis, those that signal the process, those that activate apoptosis, and those that are substrates for the apoptotic pathway (Wang, 1997). Underexpression of apoptosis will increase cell survival, and this is important in cancer development (Thatte and Dahanukar, 1997). On the other hand, overexpression of apoptosis will result in excess cell death, which may be of relevance in SMA and ALS. There is accumulating evidence that apoptosis, rather than necrotic nerve cell death, is a significant factor underlying ALS and other neurodegenerative diseases (Lo et al., 1995; Martin 1999, 2000). In ALS, some of the dying cells show characteristics of apoptosis. They appear pyknotic at the light and electron microscopic level, do not provoke active inflammation, and display DNA fragmentation by in situ end labeling techniques (Yoshiyama et al., 1994). Reactive oxygen species are involved in the induction and progression of apoptosis (Veis et al., 1993; Hockenbery et al., 1993), particularly in neurons (Kane et al., 1993; Troy and Shelanski, 1994; Greenlund et al., 1995). In this context, it is of great interest that the major genetic cause of ALS is a mutation in the gene encoding SOD-1 (Rose et al., 1993; Deng et al., 1993), an enzyme involved in the detoxification of reactive oxygen species (see Chapter 4).

Most recently, research into apoptosis has focused on two major families of genes, namely the Bcl-2 family (Oltvai et al., 1993; Krajewski et al., 1994; Martin, 1999) and the caspase (cysteine aspartases) family (Talanian et al., 1997; Van de Craen et al., 1997; Martin, 1999). The former genes act mainly as regulators in the cascade of death signal transduction controlling the execution of apoptosis, which is largely carried by the latter. The Bcl-2 gene was the first of the family to be discovered and is located at the break-point region of the t(14;18) chromosomal translocation, being present in up to 85% of follicular B-cell lymphomas in humans (Yin et al., 1994). Bcl-2 is a 26-KD integral membrane protein located on membranes of various intracellular structures, including mitochondria, which is now believed to be a major platform for the process of apoptosis. In many types of cells, expression of Bcl-2 prevents cell death from a variety of insults, including glutamate toxicity and reactive oxygen species-mediated damage.

Under normal conditions, members in the caspase family are often at proenzymatic status. The proteolytic activity of these enzymes can be induced by upstream elements in the death signal cascade to carry the death process to the final stage. It has been recently proposed that Bcl-2 regulates the activity of caspases by two possible mechanisms (Mignotte and Vayssiere, 1998). Firstly,

Bcl-2 may drag caspases to intracellular membranes such as the mitochondrial membrane through a protein called Apaf-1 (apoptosis protease-activating factor 1) to prevent the activation of caspases. Secondly, Bcl-2 may control the release from mitochondria of certain factors that induce apoptosis. Some of the known factors are cytochrome C and AIF (apoptosis-inducing factor). However, some members of the Bcl-2 family such as Bax and Bcl-Xs sharing a similar amino acid structure are pro-apoptotic proteins. Expression of Bax can be induced by the tumor suppressor protein p53 upon certain apoptotic stimuli and consequently results in apoptosis in many types of cells. Bcl-2 can form a hetrodimer with Bax or Bcl-Xs that may interrupt the transduction of death signal carried by Bax/Bcl-Xs (Oltvai et al., 1993). Therefore, within the Bcl-2 family, interactions between apoptosis regulators reflect an intracellular regulatory mechanism (or check-point) in the transduction of cell death signaling. Depending on the nature of a death signal, this check-point may occur quite late in the signal transduction pathway. For instance, in the case of glutamate induced cytotoxicity in cultured cortical neurons, it was shown that expressing Bcl-2 can prevent glutamate-induced apoptotic neuronal cell death as late as 8 hours after the initial glutamate insult (Jia et al., 1995; Baumgartner and Shine, 1997).

Recent research is beginning to show how specific macromolecules play a role in determining the apoptotic death process. Tatton and colleagues (1997) have studied the critical nature of gradual mitochondrial failure in the apoptotic process and proposed that mitochondrial function might be maintained through the pharmacological modulation of gene expression. Bcl-2 is able to block apoptosis in neurons by reducing the generation of reactive oxygen species (Migheli et al., 1994). Immunohistochemical expression of Bcl-2 protein in the aged brain and in various human neurodegenerative diseases is enriched within lipofuscin and autophagic vacuoles of neurons, glial, and vascular cells. Since oxidative stress is directly involved in lipofuscinogenesis, accumulation of Bcl-2 may reflect a mechanism for counterbalancing reactive oxygen species mediated damage, or it might represent the impairment of Bcl-2 dependent protection from reactive oxygen species (Migheli et al., 1994). Upregulation of Bcl-2, which could be possible through gene transfer, would then retard or even reverse apoptosis and help maintain a greater number of functioning neurons.

It has been demonstrated that deprenyl can reduce neuronal apoptosis caused by a variety of agents in different neuronal sub-types. One of the principal metabolites of deprenyl is desmethyldeprenyl, and it mediates anti-apoptotic action (Tatton et al., 1997). This is not a trivial observation, because the drug is cheap, safe, and readily available. Deprenyl induces altered expression of a number of genes in pre-apoptotic neurons. They include the genes for SOD-1 and SOD-2, Bcl-2, and Bcl-Xl, nitric oxide synthase, c-JUN, and nicotinamide adenine dinucleotide dehydrogenase. Unfortunately, the kinetics of deprenyl metabolism and its biodistribution after oral administration greatly limit its anti-apoptotic action, mitigating against potential benefit in neurodegenerative disease. This again is a problem of ineffectual delivery and may be greatly enhanced by using a transdermal patch, liposomal packaging, or eventually through use of viral vectors.

Grafting of functioning neurons into the central nervous system

The developing, and even the adult, mammalian CNS contain a population of undifferentiated, multipotent cell precursors, neural stem cells. The plastic properties of these cells offer an exciting and unique advantage in the design of more effective therapies for many neurological diseases. Multipotent neural progenitors and stem cells may integrate appropriately into the developing and degenerating central nervous system. They may also be effective in the replacement of genes, cells, and non-diffusible factors in either a widespread or a more circumscribed manner (Snyder, 1994; Snyder and Flax, 1995; Taylor, 1997; Park et al., 1999; Ourednik et al., 2000 and Akerud et al., 2001). There is a growing body of evidence to indicate that immortalized multi-potent neural progenitors can become integrated into the adult central nervous system. Is it then possible to replenish the degenerating corticomotoneurons and spinal motor neurons affected in motor neuron diseases?

Multipotential neural stem cells can potentially replace dead, degenerating or diseased neurological tissue. In contrast to renewable tissue, such as the blood, skin epithelium, or immune system, which have specialized, self-renewing cells known as stem cells, it has been generally argued that mammalian CNS precursor cells, if they exist, only have a very limited proliferative or lineage potential ceasing before or shortly after birth. (Weiss et al., 1996). Findings over the past decade have clearly proven that this is incorrect and that new neurons continue to be added into the brains of adult fish, frogs, reptiles, birds, and mammals (Alvarez-Buylla et al., 1995). The persistent neurogenesis in the adult brain, which is a possible endogenous repair program, may underlie cellular plasticity in the adult brain in response to environmental stimuli and injury and raises hopes for novel approaches to brain repair. By understanding the mechanisms involved, it may be possible to harness this plasticity to recruit endogenous neural stem cells or to graft stem cells to achieve structural brain repair (Peterson, 2002). The precursor cells giving rise to the neurons generated in adulthood are generally located in the walls of the brain ventricles. From here, the neuronal precursors can migrate and are capable of traversing to distant sites where they are able to differentiate into a variety of neurons and glia.

Neuronal precursors can be induced to proliferate in vitro when exposed to growth factors and retain their potential to differentiate into neurons and glia. The neuronal precursors of the adult brain could then be used as a source of cells for neuronal transplantation (Brustle and McKay, 1996). Cells can be isolated from the brain of various species, including human fetal and adult operative tissue, and can be maintained in an undifferentiated state in vitro in the presence of epidermal growth factor. After removing the epidermal growth factor, the cells cease mitosis and can be induced to differentiate into neurons, astrocytes, and oligodendrocytes, which can then be injected into different neural structures (Hammang et al., 1997). For example, when stem cells are injected into a myelin-deficient rat spinal cord, they respond to cues within the mutant CNS and differentiate into myelinating oligodendrocytes (Hammang et al., 1997).

On transplantation into the host brain, the progenitor cells can differentiate into functioning neurons and glia in response to local micro-environmental signals (Snyder, 1994; Snyder and Flax, 1995). Unlike fetal neural tissue, which is difficult to obtain and ethically problematic, the inherent biological properties of neural progenitors grown in tissue culture make them ideal for cell replacement. These cells can also be used as vehicles for gene and drug delivery. Snyder (1995) has demonstrated the feasibility of successful gene transfer throughout the CNS, including the ability to replete lost or dysfunctional neural populations. Targeted photolytic cell death is a technique which can experimentally eliminate sub-populations of neurons and provides a highly controllable model of neuronal degeneration in the adult CNS (Macklis, 1993). The cell death induced is apoptotic, not necrotic, and has the potential of creating a microenvironment that might recapitulate the signals mediated by apoptosis during normal development. This would allow transplanted progenitor cells to respond by differentiating into normal functioning neurons. When neural progenitors are transplanted into adult mouse cortex within the regions of photolytic degeneration, they do in fact differentiate into pyramidal neurons, replacing the degenerated population (Snyder and Flax, 1995). Because neural progenitors are influenced to divide using growth factors, rather than oncogenes, and because they appear to make appropriate lineage decisions when transplanted into a mutant environment, they may provide an excellent source of cells for a variety of future therapies using cellular transplantation (Martinez-Serrano and Byorklund, 1995–96; Snyder and Macklis, 1995–96; Snyder et al., 1997). Ultimately, it may become possible to derive stem cells from human umbilical cord blood or even adult venous blood that are capable of differentiating into neurons. In a very recent experiment it was shown that *SOD1* mutant mice injected with human umbilical cord blood cells lived about nine days longer and developed symptoms eleven days later than control animals (Kalkanis et al., 2001).

Ongoing experiments in both rodents and primates have shown that it is feasible and safe to inject neuronal precursors in the spinal cord of normal animals and *SOD1* mutants (Snyder EY, personal communication). This has been done with a view to treating ALS. It is unknown to what extent cells injected into the spinal cord migrate, and present thinking would dictate that injections would have to be made at several spinal levels. This is not an undertaking that could be readily considered in humans with ALS. There would be considerable danger of spinal cord damage. Clearly, it would be much easier to transplant neural progenitors into a circumscribed region such as the motor cortex than into the whole spinal cord. This raises the question of how important is the motor cortex in the etiopathogenesis of ALS. Eisen et al. (1992; 1995; 1997; 1998) have proposed that ALS might even originate in the motor cortex, the concept originally proposed by Charcot (Charcot, 1865; Charcot and Joffroy, 1869). Others would disagree and argue that the disease commences in the spinal motor neurons, spreading retrogradely to the upper motor neurons (Chou and Norris, 1993), or affects both the upper and lower motor neurons independently of each other (Kiernan and Hudson, 1991; Pamphlett et al., 1995; Chou et al., 1996). Whichever of these views proves to be correct, the corticomotoneuronal system in humans is unique and greatly expanded at the expense of other descending tracts. The cells of origin of the cortico-motoneuronal system are amongst the largest in the nervous system and include the Betz cells, and injecting stem cells into the motor cortex would be relatively straightforward. Their large size makes them particularly vulnerable to excitotoxic and oxidative stresses and they play an essential role in the ALS degenerative process (Mann, 1994). The same holds true for SMA since spinal motor neurons and their extensions are equally large and vulnerable to a variety of internal and external environmental stresses.

Future pharmacotherapy

Pharmacogenomics is the application of genomic technologies such as gene sequencing, statistical genetics, and gene expression analysis to drugs. Genomics, particularly high-throughput sequencing and characterization of expressed human genes, has created new opportunities for drug discovery (Emilien et al., 2000). Knowledge of all the human genes and their functions will allow much more effective preventive measures and will change drug research strategy and drug discovery processes. The potential implication of genomics and pharma-cogenomics in clinical research and clinical medicine is that disease could be treated according to genetic and specific individual markers; medication selection and dosages could be optimized for individual patients. The possibility of defining patient populations genetically may improve outcomes by predicting individual responses to drugs and could improve safety and efficacy in therapeutic areas such as neurodegenerative disease. However, there are important ethical issues that first must be addressed before the use of genomics in clinical research and clinical medicine.

In summary, gene-mediated therapy will open avenues to protect the aging genome, modify apoptosis (a reversible mechanism of neuronal death), and enhance drug delivery especially for neurotrophic factors. Injection of neural progenitor cells that could replenish dying and dead neurons is potenitally the most exciting future avenue. Progenitor cell transfer can also be adopted as a therapeutic vehicle. The future for treating ALS and SMA looks encouraging.

References

Aebischer P, Pochon NA, Heyd B, Deglon N et al. (1996) Gene therapy for amyotrophic lateral sclerosis (ALS) using a polymer encapsulated xenogenic cell line engineered to secrete rhCNTF. Human Gene Therapy 7:851–860.

Aisner DL, Wright WE, Shay JW (2002) Telomerase regulation: not just flipping the switch. Curr Opin Genet Dev 12:80–85.

Akerud P, Canals JM, Snyder EY, Arenas E (2001) Neuroprotection through delivery of glial cell line-derived neurotrophic factor by neural stem cells in a mouse model of Parkinson's disease. J Neurosci 21:8108–8118.

Al-Chalabi A, Powell JF, Leigh PN (1995) Neurofilaments, free radicals, excitotoxins and amyotrophic lateral sclerosis. Muscle & Nerve 18:540–545.

Alvarez-Buylla A, Lois C (1995) Neuronal stem cells in the brain of adult vertebrates. Stem cells 13:263–272.

Apfel SC (2002) Is the therapeutic application of neurotrophic factors dead? Ann Neurol 51:8–11.

Ascadi G, Anguelov R, Lewis RA, Jani A, Yang H et al. (2001) C67 adenoviral mediated GDNF gene transfer in SOD-1 mice. ALS 2 (Suppl 2) Pp 46.

Baumgartner, BJ, Shine HD (1997) Targeted transduction of CNS neurons with adenoviral vectors carrying neurotrophic factor genes confers neuroprotection that exceeds the transduced population. J Neurosci 17:6504–6511.

Baynes JW (2000) From life to death—the struggle between chemistry and biology during aging: the Maillard reaction as an amplifier of genomic damage. Biogerontology 1(3):235–246.

Beal F (1995) Aging, energy, and oxidative stress in neurodegenerative diseases. Ann Neurol 38:357–366.

Bilang BA, Revah F, Colin P, Locquet I et al. (1997) Intrastriatal injection of an adenoviral vector expressing glial-cell-line-derived neurotrophic factor prevents dopaminergic neuron degeneration and behavioral impairment in a rat model of Parkinson disease. Proc Natl Acad Sci USA 94:8818–8823.

Brauner R, Nonoyama M, Laks H, Drinkwater DJ et al. (1997) Intracoronary adenovirus-mediated transfer of immunosuppressive cytokine genes prolongs allograft survival. J Thorac Cardiovasc Surg. 114:923–933.

Brustle O, McKay RD (1996) Neuronal progenitors as tools for cell replacement in the nervous system. Current Opinion in Neurobiology 6:688–695.

Brzustowicz LM, Lehner T, Castilla H et al. (1990) Genetic mapping of chronic childhood-onset spinal muscular atrophy to chromosome 5q11.2–13.3 Nature 344:540–541.

Bui LA, Butterfield LH, Kim JY et al. (1997) In vivo therapy of hepatocellular carcinoma with a tumor-specific adenoviral vector expressing interleukin-2. Hum Gene Ther 8:2173–2182.

Charcot JM (1865) Sclerose des cordons lateraux de la moelle epinere chez femme hysterique atteinte de contracture peranemte des quatre membres. Bull Soc Med Hop Paris 2(suppl 2):24–42.

Charcot JM, Joffroy A (1869) Deux cas d'atrophie musculaire progressive avec lesions de la substance grise et des faisceaux anterolateraux de la moelle epiniere. Arch Physiol Norm Pathol; 2:354–367, 629–649, 744–760.

Chou SM, Norris FH (1993) Amyotrophic lateral sclerosis: lower motor neuron disease spreading to upper motor neurons. Muscle & Nerve; 16:864–869.

Chou SM, Wang HS, Komai K (1996) Colocalization of NOS and SODI in neurofilament accumulation within the motor neurons of amyotrophic lateral sclerosis: an immunohistochemical study. J Chem Neuroanat 10:249–258.

Corcia P, Mayeux-Portas V, Khoris J et al. (2002) Abnormal SMN1 gene copy number is a susceptibility factor for amyotrophic lateral sclerosis. Ann Neurol. 51:243–6.

Cortopassi GA, Wang E (1996) There is substantial agreement among interspecies estimates of DNA repair activity. Mechanisms of Ageing & Development 91:211–218.

Counter CM, Meyerson M, Eaton EN, Ellisen LW et al. (1998) Telomerase activity is restored in human cells by ectopic expression of hTERT (hEST2), the catalytic subunit of telomerase. Oncogene 16:1217–1222.

Crawford TO (1996) From enigmatic to problematic: The new molecular genetics of childhood spinal muscular atrophy. Neurology 46:335–340.

Dahse R, Fiedler W, Ernst G (1997) Telomeres and telomerase: biological and clinical importance. Clin Chem 43:708–714.

Davidson BL, Bohn MC (1997) Recombinant adenovirus: a gene transfer vector for study and treatment of CNS diseases. Exp Neurol 144:125–130.

Deng H-X, Hentati A, Tainer JA et al. (1993) Amyotrophic lateral sclerosis and structural defects in Cu, Zn superoxide dismutase. Science 261:1047–1051.

Eisen A, Kim S, Pant B (1992) Amyotrophic lateral sclerosis (ALS): a phylogenetic disease of the corticomotoneuron? Muscle & Nerve 15:219–228.

Eisen A (1995) Amyotrophic lateral sclerosis is a multifactorial disease. Muscle & Nerve 18:741–752.

Eisen A, Nakajima M, Enterzari-Taher M, Stewart H (1997) The corticomotoneuron: aging, sporadic amyotrophic lateral sclerosis (ALS) and first degree relatives. In: Physiology of ALS and related diseases. Kimura J, Kaji R (eds). Elsevier Science, Holland., pp155–175.

Eisen A, Krieger C (1998) Amyotrophic Lateral Sclerosis: A Synthesis of Research and Clinical Practice. Cambridge University Press, UK.

Emilien G, Ponchon M, Caldas C, Isacson O, Maloteaux JM (2000) Impact of genomics on drug discovery and clinical medicine. QJM; 93:391–423.

Emtage PC, Wan Y, Bramson JL, Graham FL and Gauldie J (1998) A double recombinant adenovirus expressing the costimulatory molecule B7-1 (murine) and human IL-2 induces complete tumor regression in a murine breast adenocarcinoma model. J Immunol 160:2531–2538.

Felgner JH, Kumar R, Sridhar CN, Wheeler CJ, Tsai YJ, Border R, Ramsey P, Martin M and Felgner PL (1994) Enhanced gene delivery and mechanism studies with a novel series of cationic lipid formulations. Journal of Biological Chemistry 269:2550–2561.

Felzmann T, Ramsey WJ and Blaese RM (1997) Characterization of the antitumor immune response generated by treatment of murine tumors with recombinant adenoviruses expressing HSVtk, IL-2, IL-6 or B7-1. Gene Ther 4:1322–1329.

Figlewicz DA, Krizus A, Martinoli MG et al. (1994) Variants of the heavy neruofilament subunit are associated with development of amyotrophic lateral sclerosis. Hum Mol Genet 3:1757–1761.

Fisher LJ, Ray J (1994) In vivo and ex vivo gene transfer to the brain. Curr Opinion Neurobiol; 4:735–741.

Ghavami A, Baruscotti M, Robinson RB and Hen R (1997) Adenovirus-mediated expression of 5-HT1B receptors in cardiac ventricle myocytes; coupling to inwardly rectifying K+ channels. Eur J Pharmacol 340: 259–266.

Gimenez Y, Ribotta M, Revah F, Pradier L et al. (1997) Prevention of motoneuron death by adenovirus-mediated neurotrophic factors. Journal of Neuroscience Research. 48:281–285.

Glorioso JC, Goins WF, Fink DJ and DeLuca NA (1994) Herpes simplex virus vectors and gene transfer to brain. Developments in Biological Standardization 82:79–87.

Gravel C, Gotz R, Lorrain A and Sendtner M (1997) Adenoviral gene transfer of ciliary neurotrophic factor and brain-derived neurotrophic factor leads to long-term survival of axotomized motor neurons. Nat Med 3:765–770.

Greenlund LJS, Deckwerth TL, Johnson EM (1995) Superoxide dismutase delays neuronal apoptosis: a role for reactive oxygen species in programmed neuronal death. Neuron 14:303–315.

Greider CW (1998) Telomeres and senescence: the history, the experiment, the future. Current Biol 8:178–181.

Gunzburg WH, Fleuchaus A, Saller R and Salmons B (1996) Retroviral vector targeting for gene therapy. Cytokines Mol Ther 2:177–184.

Haase G, Kennel P, Pettmann B, Vigne E et al. (1997) Gene therapy of murine motor neuron disease using adenoviral vectors for neurotrophic factors. Nature Med 3:429–436.

Hammang JP, Archer DR, Duncan ID (1997) Myelination following transplantation of EGF-responsive neural stem cells into a myelin deficient environment. Experimental Neurol 147:84–95.

Harley CB (1997) Human aging and telomeres. Ciba Foundation Symposium 211:129–139.

Harley CB, Sherwood SW (1997) Telomerase, checkpoints and cancer. Cancer Surveys 29:263–284.

Hockenbery DM, Oltvai ZN, Yin X-M, Milliman CL, Korsmeyer SJ (1993) Bcl-2 functions in an antioxidant pathway to prevent apoptosis. Cell 75:241–251.

Horellou, P and Mallet J (1997) Gene therapy for Parkinson's disease. Mol Neurobiol 15:241–256.

Hughes SM, Moussavi-Harami F, Sauter SL, Davidson BL (2002) Viral-mediated gene transfer to mouse primary neural progenitor cells. Mol Ther 5:16–24.

Ince P, Stout N, Shaw P, Slade J et al. (1993) Parvalbumin and calbindin D-28k in the human motor system in motor neuron disease. Neuropath & Appl Neurobiol 19:291–299.

Jia W (1995) A bcl-2 viral vector protects neurons from excitoxicity even when administrated several hours after the toxic insult. Neurosci pp. 21: 72.

Johns DR (1996) The other human genome: mitochondrial DNA and disease. Nature Medicine 2:1065–1068.

Julien JP (1995) A role for neurofilaments in the pathogenesis of amyotrophic lateral sclerosis. Biochem Cell Biol 73:593–597.

Kaal EC, Joosten EA, Bar PR (1997) Prevention of apoptotic motoneuron death in vitro by neurotrophins and muscle extract. Neurochemistry International 31:193–201.

Kalkanis SN, Dreibelbiss J, Welty C, Haque J, et al. (2001) C6 stem cell transplantation delays onset, improves survival in transgenic ALS mice. ALS 2: (Suppl 2) Pp5.

Kane DJ, Sarafian TA, Anton R, Hahn H et al. (1993) Bcl-2 inhibition of neural death: Decreased generationof reactive oxygen species. Science 262:1274–1277.

Kasahara N, Dozy AM, Kan YW (1994) Tissue-specific targeting of retroviral vectors through ligand-receptor interactions. Science; 266:1373–1376.

Kay MA, Woo SLC (1994) Gene therapy for metabolic disorders. Trends Genet; 10:253–257.

Kiernan JA, Hudson AJ (1991) Changes in sizes of cortical and lower motor neurons in amyotrophic lateral sclerosis. Brain; 114:843–853.

Krajewski S, Krajewska M, Shabaik A, Miyashita T et al. (1994) Immunohistochemical determination of in vivo distribution of Bax, a dominant inhibitor of Bcl-2. American Journal of Pathology 145:1323–1336.

Kruk PA, Balajee AS, Rao KS, Bohr VA (1996) Telomere reduction and telomerase inactivation during neuronal cell differentiation. Biochem Biophys Res Commun 224:487–492.

Landman J, Kavaler E, Droller, Liu BC (1997) Applications of telomerase in urologic oncology. World J Urol 15:120–124.

Liu F, Huang L (2002) Development of non-viral vectors for systemic gene delivery. J Control Release 78:259–266.

Lo AC, Houenou LJ, Oppenheim RW (1995) Apoptosis in the nervous system: morphological features, methods, pathology, and prevention. Archives of Histology & Cytology 58:139–149.

Macklis JD (1993) Transplanted neocortical neurons migrate selectively into regions of neuronal degeneration produced by chromophore-targeted laser photolysis. J Neurosci 13:3848–3863.

Mallet J (1996) The TiPS/TINS Lecture. Catecholamines: from gene regulation to neuropsychiatric disorders. Trends Neurosci 19:191–196.

Mann DM (1994) Vulnerability of specific neurons to aging. In: Neurodegenerative Diseases, Calne DB (Ed), WB Saunders CO, Philadelphia, pp15–31.

Martin LJ (1999) Neuronal death in amyotrophic lateral sclerosis is apoptosis: possible contribution of a programmed cell death mechanism. J Neuropathol Exp Neurol 58:459–471.

Martin LJ (2000) p53 is abnormally elevated and active in the CNS of patients with amyotrophic lateral sclerosis. Neurobiol Dis 7:613–622.

Martinez-Serrano A, Bjorklund A (1995) Gene transfer to the mammalian brain using neural stem cells: a focus on trophic factors, neurodegeneration, and cholinergic neuron systems. Clinical Neurosci 3:301–309.

McClearn GE (1997) Prospects for quantitative trait locus methodology in gerontology. Experimental Gerontology 32:49–54.

Melki J, Abdelhak S, Sheth P et al. (1990) Gene for chronic proximal spinal muscular atrophies maps to chromosome 5q. Nature 344:767–768.

Migheli A, Cavalla P, Piva R, Giordana MT, Schiffer D (1994) bcl-2 protein expression in aged brain and neurodegenerative diseases. Neuroreport 5:1906–1908.

Mignotte B and JL Vayssiere (1998) Mitochondria and apoptosis. Eur J Biochem 252:1–15.

Miller RG, Petajan JH, Bryan WW (1996) A placebo-controlled trial of recombinant human ciliary neurotrophic (rh CNTF) factor in amyotrophic lateral sclerosis. Ann Neurol 39:256–260.

Morin GB (1997) Telomere control and replicative lifespan. Exp Geront 32:375–382.

Morrison BM, Janssen WG, Gordon JW, Morrison JH (1998) Time course of neuropathology in the spinal cord of G86R superoxide dismutase transgenic mice. J Comp Neurol 391:64–77.

Morrison KE (1996) Advances in SMA research: review of gene deletions. Neuromusc Disord 6:397–408.

Moulard B, Salachas F, Chassande B, et al (1998) Association between centromeric deletions of the SMN gene and sporadic adult-onset lower motor neuron disease. Ann Neurol 43:640–4.

Murphy AN, Bredesen DE, Cortopassi G, Wang E (1996) Fiskum G. Bcl-2 potentiates the maximal calcium uptake capacity of neural cell mitochondria. Proc Nat Acad Sci 93:9893–9898.

Nasz I, Adam E (2001) Recombinant adenovirus vectors for gene therapy and clinical trials Acta Microbiol Immunol 48:323–348.

O'Connor WM, Davidson BL, Kaplitt MG, Abbey MV et al. (1997) Adenovirus vector-mediated gene transfer into human epileptogenic brain slices: prospects for gene therapy in epilepsy. Exp Neurol 148:167–178.

Ohashi T, Watabe K, Uehara K, Sly WS, Vogler C and Eto Y (1997) Adenovirus-mediated gene transfer and expression of human beta- glucuronidase gene in the liver, spleen, and central nervous system in mucopolysaccharidosis type VII mice. Proc Natl Acad Sci USA. 94:1287–1292.

Oltvai ZN, Milliman CL and Korsmeyer SJ (1993) Bcl-2 heterodimerizes in vivo with a conserved homolog, Bax, that accelerates programmed cell death. Cell 74:609–619.

Ourednik V, Ourednik J, Park KI, Teng YD, Aboody KA, Auguste KI, Taylor RM, Tate BA, Snyder EY. (2000) Neural stem cells are uniquely suited for cell replacement and gene therapy in the CNS. Novartis Found Symp 231:242–262.

Park KI, Liu S, Flax JD, Nissim S, Stieg PE, Snyder EY (1999) Transplantation of neural progenitor and stem cells: developmental insights may suggest new therapies for spinal cord and other CNS dysfunction. J Neurotrauma 16:675–687.

Pamphlett R, Kril J, Hng TM (1995) Motor neuron disease: A primary disorder of corticomotoneuron? Muscle & Nerve 18:314–318.

Peltekian E, Parrish E, Bouchard C, Peschanski M, Lisovoski F (1997) Adenovirus-mediated gene transfer to the brain: methodological assessment. Journal of Neuroscience Methods 71:77–84.

Peterson DA (2002) Stem cells in brain plasticity and repair. Curr Opin Pharmacol 2:34–42.

Puyal C, Milhaud P, Bienvenue A and Philippot JR (1995) A new cationic liposome encapsulating genetic material. A potential delivery system for polynucleotides. European Journal of Biochemistry 228:697–703.

Radunovic A, Leigh PN (1996) Cu/Zn superoxide dismutase gene mutations in amyotrophic lateral sclerosis: correlation between genotype and clinical features. J Neurol Neurosurg Psychiatry 61:565–572.

Rattan SI (1995) Ageing – a biological perspective. Molecular Aspects of Med 16:439–508.

Robbins PD, Tahara H and Ghivizzani SC (1998) Viral vectors for gene therapy. Trends Biotechnol 16:35–40.

Roizman B (1996) The function of herpes simplex virus genes: a primer for genetic engineering of novel vectors. Proceedings of the National Academy of Sciences of the United States of America 93:11307–11312.

Rose DR, Siddique T, Patterson D, Figlewicz DA et al. (1993) Mutations in Cu/Zn superoxide dismuate gene are associated with familial amyotrophic lateral sclerosis. Nature 362:59–62.

Rosenblum CI and Chen HY (1995) In ovo transfection of chicken embryos using cationic liposomes. Transgenic Research 4:192–198.

Rothstein J (1995) Excitotoxic mechanisms in the pathogenesis of amyotrophic lateral sclerosis. In: Pathogenesis and Therapy of Amyotrophic Lateral Sclerosis. Serratrice G, Munsat T (Eds), Advances in Neurology Vol 68, Lippincott-Raven Publishers, Philadelphia, pp7–20.

Roy N, Mahadevan MS, McLean M et al. (1995) The gene for neuronal apoptosis inhibitory protein is partially deleted in individuals with spinal muscular atrophy. Cell 80:167–178.

Sahenk Z, Seharaseyon J, Mendell JR, Burghes AH (1993) Gene delivery to spinal motor neurons. Brain Research 606:126–9.

Seeburger JL, Springer JE (1993) Experimental rationale for the therapeutic use of neurotrophins in amyotrophic lateral sclerosis. Expt Neurol 124:64–72.

Simonian NA, Coyle JT (1996) Oxidative stress in neurodegenerative diseases. Ann Rev Pharmacol Toxicol 36:83–106.

Snoeck HW, Tao W and Klotman ME (1997) Adeno-associated viral vectors: background and technical aspects. Exp Nephrol 5:514–520.

Snyder EY (1994) Grafting immortalized neurons to the CNS. Current Opinion in Neurology 4:742–751.

Snyder EY, Flax JD (1995) Transplantation of neural progenitor and stem-like cells as a strategy for gene therapy and repair of neurodegenerative diseases. Mental Redardation and Developmental Disabilities Research Reviews 1:27–38.

Snyder EY, Macklis JD (1995–96) Multipotential neural progenitor or stem-like cells may be uniquely suited for therapy for some neurodegenerative conditions. Clinical Neurosi 3:310–316.

Snyder EY, Park KI, Flax JD, Liu S et al. (1997) Potential of neural 'stem-like' cells for gene therapy and repair of the degenerating central nervous system. Advances in Neurol 72:121–132.

Steinert S, White DM, Zou Y, Shay JW, Wright WE (2002) Telomere biology and cellular aging in nonhuman primate cells. Exp Cell Res 272:146–152.

Sorscher EJ, Logan JJ, Frizzell RA et al. (1994) Gene therapy for cystic fibrosis using cationic liposome mediated gene transfer: a phase I trial of safety and efficacy in the nasal airway. Human Gene Therapy 5:1259–1277.

Talanian RV, Quinlan C, Trautz S et al. (1997) Substrate specificities of caspase family proteases. Journal of Biological Chemistry 272:9677–9682.

Tatton WG, Chalmers-Redman RM, Ju WY, Wadia J, Tatton NA (1997) Apoptosis in neurodegenerative disorders: potential for therapy by modifying gene transcription. Journal of Neural Transmission (Suppl). 49:245–68.

Taylor R (1997) Cell vehicles for gene transfer to the brain. Neuromuscular Disorders 7:343–351.

Thatte U, Dahanukar S (1997) Apoptosis: clinical relevance and pharmacological manipulation. Drugs 54:511–32.

Troy CM, Shelanski ML (1994) Down-regulation of copper/zinc superoxide dismutase causes apoptotic death in PC12 neuronal cells. Proc Natl Acad Sci USA 91:6384–6387.

Umegaki H, Chernak JM, Ikari H, Roth GS and Ingram DK (1997) Rotational behavior produced by adenovirus-mediated gene transfer of dopamine D2 receptor into rat striatum. Neuroreport 8: 3553–3558.

Van de Craen M, Vandenabeele P, Declercq W et al. (1997) Characterization of seven murine caspase family members. Febs Letters 403:61–69.

Vaziri H, Benchimol S (1998) Reconstitution of telomerase activity in normal human cells leads to elongation of telomeres and extended relpicative life span. Current Biol 8:279–282.

Veis DJ, Sorenson CM, Shutter JR, Korsmeyer SJ (1993) Bcl-2-deficient mice demonstrate fulminant lymphoid apoptosis, polycystic kidneys, and hypopigmented hair. Cell 75:229–240.

Veldink JH, van den Berg LH, Cobben JM et al. (2001) Homozygous deletion of the survival motor neuron 2 gene is a prognostic factor in sporadic ALS. Neurology 56:749–52.

Venter JC, Adams MD, Myers EW et al. (2001) The sequence of the human genome. Science 291:1304–1351.

Vijg J, van Orsouw N (2002) Searching for genetic determinants of human aging and longevity: opportunities and challenges. Mech Ageing Dev 123:195–205.

Wang E (1997) Regulation of apoptosis resistance and ontogeny of age-dependent diseases. Experimental Gerontology 32:471–84.

Weiss S, Reynolds BA, Vescovi AL, Morshead C et al. (1996) Is there a neural stem cell in mammalian forebrain Trends in Neurosci 19:387–393.

Yagi K, Hayashi Y, Ishida N, Ohbayashi M et al. (1994) Interferon-beta endogenously produced by intratumoral injection of cationic liposome-encapsulated gene: cytocidal effect on glioma transplanted into nude mouse brain. Biochemistry & Molecular Biology International 32:167–171.

Yanagi K, Mochida A, Gotoh E (1997) Telomere DNA and telomerase of lymphoma-derived cell lines – telomere hypothesis for cell growth control. Nippon Rinsho – Japanese J Clin Med 55:328–333.

Yin XM, Oltval ZN and Korsmeyer SJ (1994) BH1 and BH2 domains of Bcl-2 are required for inhibition of apoptosis and heterodimerization with Bax. Nature 369:321–323.

Yoshiyama Y, Yamada T, Asanma K, Ashahi T (1994) Apoptosis related antigen, Ley and nick-end labeling are positive in spinal motor neurons in amyotrophic lateral slcerosis. Acta Neuropathologica 88:207–211.

Zakian VA (1995) Telomeres: beginning to understand the end. Science 270:1601–1607.

Index

Note: page numbers in *italics* refer to figures and tables